Home Remedies Bible: Complete Guide on Your Own Home Remedies

Home Remedies to Cure Everyday Ailments

I0414271

By: Mihalis Kapakolis

9781631871658

PUBLISHERS NOTES

Speedy Publishing LLC

40 E Main Street,

Newark

Delaware

19711

Contact Us: 1-888-248-4521

Website: http://www.speedypublishing.co

REPRINTED Paperback Edition: ISBN: 9781631871658

Manufactured in the United States of America

DEDICATION

This book is dedicated to all my family and loved ones who inspired me to do the research necessary to compile this detailed guide on how to heal the body naturally using items found in the home. I also wish to dedicate this book to persons who aim to adopt a healthier lifestyle by limiting their consumption of conventional medications. I hope this book will provide the answers you need.

CONTENTS

Chapter 1- Remedies for Skin Conditions

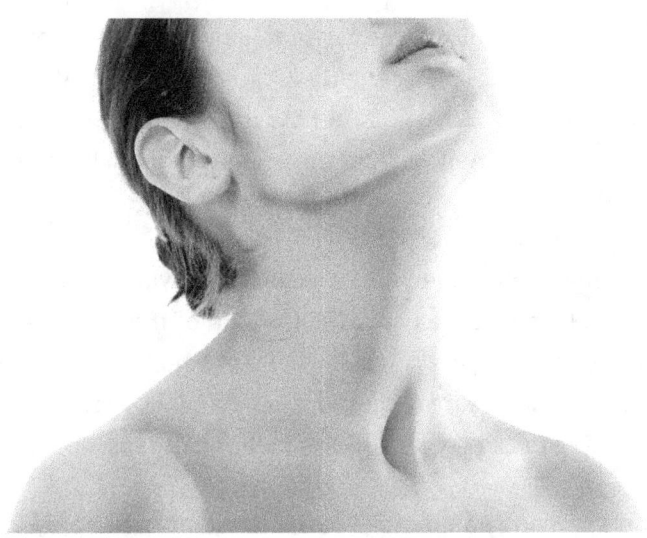

Dry Skin

When your skin is dry, home remedy skin care opportunities can really come in handy. There are many different things that you can do to improve your dry skin. The more different dry skin remedies that you pursue, the better your skin will benefit. Here is a list of some of the best home remedies for dealing with dry skin. In severe cases of dealing with dry skin, you may want to apply either avocado oil or castor oil for the skin. When it comes to situations when your skin is really dry, home remedy skin care involving the application of natural oils is typically a good way to go.

Combine together a teaspoon worth of green clay powder and a teaspoon of raw honey, and then apply this mixture, once it has been well prepared, to your face or any other area where your skin is dry. If you are applying it to your face, make sure to avoid the area around your eyes. Leave this mixture on your skin for between 15 minutes and 20 minutes, and then use lukewarm water to wash it away. This is a really simple and useful home remedy for dealing with dry skin.

Another useful dry skin treatment is actually regular exercise, believe it or not. Exercising regularly is going to improve your body's blood circulation. When blood flow is properly encouraged, then the proper nourishment will be provided to your skin in order to keep it healthy.

Another truly important remedy for dry skin is for you to avoid the consumption of alcohol as well as caffeine. Both of these things can cause dry skin, or even make it worse if you are not careful. If you consume either of these substances in excess and are dealing with dry skin, try cutting back on them and see what happens.

Another good dry skin remedy for you to consider is to apply aloe vera gel to your face and other areas where your skin is dry after bathing. After taking a warm bath, your pores will be open and much more receptive to the healing and moisturizing power of the Aloe Vera.

All of these dry skin remedies can be extremely useful on your face and other areas of your body where your skin is dry as well. You can combine different treatment options to meet your needs until you find the remedies that will best suit you. If one specific dry skin remedy is not helping your skin become more moisturized, then you should move onto the next one until you find something that is definitely giving you the results that you are looking for.

There are a wide variety of natural ways to improve your skin. Dry skin isn't doing you any favors, so make a point to improve your skin sooner rather than later.

BOILS

Mihalis Kapakolis

Boils are caused by an infection that enters the skin through a cut or tear of the skin. At first they will be fairly small and red, as the infection progresses the boil will fill with pus and get bigger and start to look more white than red. Once the boil has gotten to this point there are some things you can do to help get rid of it safely. Here is an easy to use boil home remedy.

Boils can show up anywhere on the skin but are usually found on the shoulders, face, groin, buttocks and thighs. They will usually last around 10 days and unless you have any underlying health issues can usually be dealt with right at home.

1. To help the boil come to a head, so that it can drain, you can use a washcloth soaked in warm water to make a compress. Apply this compress to the boil several times throughout the day. Leave it on the boil long enough to heat the skin of the boil to help draw the pus to the surface. Be careful that you check the temperature of the compress before applying it to your skin; you don't want to add insult to injury by burning yourself.

2. You can use cornmeal to make a paste to apply to the boil which will do the same thing as a warm compress, bring the boil to a head. Just mix about one half cup of water to a boil, add the cornmeal and mix it to form a paste. Apply the paste to the boil and cover with a warm washcloth. Do this several times during the day to help the boil drain more quickly.

There are other home remedies which may work but these are the two most common and the two that seem to have the highest success rate.

Additional tips to keep in mind:

1. Thoroughly wash your hands before and after you touch your boil. If you don't, you may spread the infection to others in your household or to other parts of your body.
2. If your boil is accompanied by fever or severe pain, make sure to see your doctor right away; don't wait for it to come to a head on its own.
3. If there are several boils in one area this is a sign of a more serious infection and you should see your doctor right away.
4. Make sure that you carefully wash all the washcloths and clothing that comes into contact with the boil so you don't spread the infection.
5. When the boil has drained you want to keep the area covered with antibacterial cream and a bandage to protect the new skin that is forming and to prevent Re-infection.
6. Last but not least, do not try to pop, or lance, the boil yourself. This can make the infection worse and should only be done by your doctor in a sterile environment.

Boils are a common, if gross, thing to occur. They can be painful and they are definitely unsightly but for the most part they aren't dangerous if you care for them properly. Follow this boil home remedy advice and you can get rid of your next boil more quickly and without the risk of further infection.

This recommendation is not medical advice and should not be used to replace professional medical advice from your personal medical doctor.

ECZEMA

You can relieve a lot of your suffering by finding an herbal remedy for eczema. If you are like the thousands of other people who have to live with eczema for the rest of their lives, you have probably found that prescribed medications don't work.

Mihalis Kapakolis

Over the counter treatments may also be ineffective, because honestly everyone's eczema is a little bit different. You might not even want to have to deal with the chemicals anyway because they can have negative side effects. The truth is that sometimes nature is the best way to treat a disease.

Many plants found in nature have healing qualities and you have a lot to choose from. You can mix and match herbal ointments and combine them in a variety of ways to create the best treatment for you. You may have to play around with a bunch of different mixtures until you find what works the best.

Aloe Vera is a plant substance that has many healing qualities. It is often used to safely relieve itching and it works well for eczema inflammation too. You can find the extract of the plant, or to go completely natural, grow one in your home. The inside of the leaves is what has the healing power when directly applied to the skin.

Witch Hazel is an uncommon herbal remedy that most people don't know about. However, it has been an anti-inflammatory treatment used by mothers who had the idea passed down over the generations.

You can use chamomile combined with either of these two herbs to relieve the itching. Together, the three ingredients can stop the itching and the inflammation. If you combine it with a natural moisturizer such as coconut oil, you'll have a winning solution.

When you make your all natural remedy, you have to combine the ingredients into something that will allow you to apply it onto your skin. Olive oil makes a great base for herbal ingredients and you can make oil that your skin will absorb quickly.

An unscented lotion can also be used if combined with extracts of the herbs you want to use. Cocoa butter is a great choice because it adds extra moisturizing qualities and is more natural than some other types of lotion.

Herbal remedies that you can use for treating eczema go beyond what you can apply to your skin. Some people will notice a change in the appearance of their symptoms when they change the foods they eat. When the body is healthier overall, it has an easier time dealing with diseases that is might otherwise not be able to. Try adding extra vitamins and minerals to your diet by eating more fruits and vegetables. Ideally you want hearty natural foods like mangos, apples, avocado, and asparagus.

You won't always be able to make your eczema symptoms go away, but by trying natural remedies you are taking a safe route to eczema relief. Let an herbal remedy for eczema be your ticket to a life that isn't controlled by an unwanted disease.

TREATING ECZEMA WITH HERBAL REMEDIES

Back in ancient times we didn't have the modern medicine that we have today. All people had to treat their ailments were herbal remedies. In time pharmaceuticals were created replacing many herbal remedies and these became more and more popular. At one point it was only 'new age' people that used herbal treatments.

Now things are changing and people are seeking out herbal remedies again. Eczema is one condition that people look for natural treatments. There are a number of eczema herbal remedy solutions that can help to treat the symptoms of the condition.

Mihalis Kapakolis

There is no cure for eczema and this is one reason that people search for eczema herbal remedy solutions. The other reason is that pharmaceutical medicines can be quite expensive for an ongoing condition. Many prescribed creams or medicines don't have much effect on eczema and even when they do it isn't long before the symptoms return.

Although herbal treatments are not a cure for eczema they are quite effective at treating the symptoms. Symptoms of eczema include rash, dry skin, flaking or scaly skin and itching. There are dozens of different eczema herbal remedy solutions and you may need to try a few to find one that works well for you.

There are many herbal or health stores that will sell the herbs needed for these remedies. You can also find online stores that will stock the herbs that you are looking for. There are never any shortages of the effective herbs for treating this condition.

Some herbal remedies for eczema will require that you make a paste with the herbs and then apply the paste to the affected areas. Some remedies require eating the herbs to gain the benefits from them.

So what types of herbs are helpful in treating eczema? Let's take a look at some useful herbs and in some cases a combination of herbs works well.

Aloe is one herb that is very effective for many skin conditions. Aloe is found in many moisturizing creams and works by moisturizing the skin. Dry skin is one of the symptoms of eczema and the aloe works well to counter the dry skin.

Calendula herb is also very good when made into a cream and applied to the skin. This will soothe the skin so it is particularly good for skin that is red and inflamed. Oregon grape root and witch hazel are two other herbs that work in a similar way.

Another good eczema herbal remedy solution is to add rosemary to your bath water. Rosemary will help stimulate circulation in the skin which will assist with healing. Oat straw is another herb that will give similar results.

Chickweed or turmeric can be used in poultices and applied to the affected skin areas. This will help the skin to heal and will also relieve the pain and itching cause by eczema.

People have different triggers for their eczema and people will respond differently to treatments. A treatment that works for one person will not necessarily work for you so it is a matter of trial and error and you will soon find the right eczema herbal remedy solution that works for you.

FINDING A NATURAL REMEDY FOR ECZEMA

Eczema (also known as dermatitis) is an annoying and potentially painful disorder that affects many people around the world. Those with eczema develop rashes and suffer from severe itching on various different parts of their bodies. Unfortunately, there is no cure for it, but there are many ways to try and manage it.

In today's world, many people put a lot more stock in natural remedies for eczema and similar disorders. People have been using home-brewed remedies to help manage eczema for a long time, and many of these remedies are actually quite effective at dealing with symptoms of the disorder.

Since eczema most commonly affects young children, a natural remedy for eczema is often preferred to avoid exposing the child to harsh pharmaceuticals with nasty side effects. The natural remedy chosen may depend on the severity of the condition.

One of the best reported home remedies for eczema is simply to make changes to one's overall lifestyle. These changes include changing to a healthier diet, reducing stress, and removing potential irritants from the environments.

A healthier diet means eliminating bad snack foods that are full of nothing but sugars and other unhealthy ingredients. Reducing stress can be a more difficult thing to do, especially for children. However, there are ways to learn how to better deal with stress and they may reduce eczema symptoms.

There are other natural preventative methods that can help a person deal with eczema. Using coconut oil or other natural moisturizers can help the skin stay soft and supple. This can help to control eczema symptoms.

While that is a more long term natural cure of eczema, sometimes people are just looking for some form of immediate fix. Maybe their itching is simply driving them crazy, or their child has been itching so much that the affected areas are starting to bleed.

There are many different remedies based on herbs and other natural ingredients that can provide quick eczema relief. You may have some of these ingredients in your own home, or you may need to find some sort of specialty store to obtain them.

Perhaps the simplest natural fix for eczema is to simply apply a cold compress or similar sort of water treatment. While very basic, they can be effective at controlling the irritation caused by eczema anywhere on the body.

You can also combine a little bit of nutmeg with the water to make a paste that will help to reduce dermatitis symptoms.

Another natural remedy for eczema symptoms involves making a paste from the herbs camphor and sandalwood. Applying this paste to areas affected by eczema can result in quick relief from the itching and rash.

In addition to making your own pastes and salves from herbal compounds, you can also use herbal-based soaps to help control eczema symptoms. You can find these at many stores that specialize in natural foods and products.

It's important to remember that while eczema can't be cured, many people live almost symptom free. It's just a matter of finding the right remedy for you.

REMEDIES FOR BABY ECZEMA

If your baby is suffering from eczema, you know how uncomfortable the itchy and dry skin can be, not to mention the sore spots. Since eczema usually goes hand in hand with sensitive skin, treating it can be a bit of a challenge. Thankfully there are quite a few home remedies for baby eczema you can try.

Mihalis Kapakolis
Moisturize

Keeping baby's skin well moisturized should always be the first step in any eczema treatment. Use a natural aloe Vera lotion several times a day, especially after bathing baby. Reapply as often as need to keep baby's skin from drying out. Avoid any harsh cleansers and make sure baby is getting plenty to drink to moisturize from the inside out as well. Incidentally breastfed babies experience fewer and milder episodes of eczema.

Oatmeal Bath

When baby's skin gets very itchy, an oatmeal bath can be very soothing and help skin heal. Put two cups of oats in a food processor (or use a coffee grinder) and grind them into a powder. Add the oatmeal powder to a running bath of warm (not hot) water and stir well. Soak in the oatmeal bath for 15 minutes, rinse with clean water and dab the skin dry with a soft towel. When baby's eczema breakouts are bad, it is safe to sooth them with an oatmeal bath twice daily.

Natural Skin Wash

As mentioned above, you want to avoid any harsh skin care for baby. The following natural skin wash is very gently and helps with the itch. Combine 1 tsp of comfrey root, 1 tsp of white oak bark, 1 tsp of slippery elm bark and two cups of water in a bowl. Mix well, and then pour it into a pot; heat over medium heat until it comes to a boil, and then simmer for thirty minutes. Allow the mixture to cool, then strain out the solids and use the liquid like any face wash.

While this mixture may not completely clear up baby's eczema, it is a natural, gentle and effective cleanser that will help reduce the itching and inflammation.

When eczema really flares up, you want to get baby's skin healed back up as soon as possible. Healing lotions can help shorten the healing time and moisturize and protect your skin from future outbreaks at the same time.

Lotions to look for ate those made with blueberry leaves. Blueberry leaves are very good at relieving the inflammation of eczema and at improving the irritation that accompanies itching.

Zinc is another great ingredient. Apply zinc lotion directly on the affected area. Zinc can also be taken as a supplement in pills. Taking regularly, it can be an effective eczema treatment.

To help heal the skin, use a lotion containing vitamin E, or apply vitamin E oil directly on the affected area. It will quickly reduce itching and improve healing. Continue applying the vitamin E oil until the skin is healed.

This article is provided for information purposes only. Please consult your baby's health care provider before trying home remedies.

MOLES, WARTS AND SKIN TAGS

Some individuals are scared of surgical methods in removing moles, warts, and skin tags but they want to remove the skin lesions as they pose cosmetic problems. If you have unsightly moles, warts, and skin tags, there is no need to be scared of some acids, knife, or surgical methods. You don't have to resort to these options immediately because there are effective home methods that you can use.

The skin lesions are caused by specific viruses which produce bumps commonly on the soles of the feet, the hands, knees, and sometimes even on the face. For those who don't like the expensive surgical procedures, you can try these remedies at home to rid your skin of these unsightly skin lesions.

1. Put warm water on a small basin and soak the affected area for fifteen to 20 minutes. Dry the affected area and use a cotton ball to apply apple cider or white vinegar and leave it on for the next fifteen minutes. Wash it off and then pat dry.
2. Dissolve aspirin with a drop of water. Apply the solution to the affected area and cover it with plaster or ban aid. Do this twice every day.
3. Baking soda and a bit of water can be rubbed over the affected area 3 to 4 times each day. For moles, soak gauge cloth with castor oil and baking soda and place it over the mole. Leave it on overnight.
4. Plantar warts are quite painful. You can use banana peel to treat it but it could take months before you can remove the warts. Do this every day and remove it only when you take a bath.
5. If you have cashew nuts at home, chew it first and place it over the affected area. Do this for a month and the skin lesions will disappear.
6. Warts can be rubbed with the open stem of dandelion. Repeat this procedure for 3 times in day.
7. Crushed garlic is also one effective way of removing warts. Secure the crushed garlic pulp with a plaster or band aid overnight.
8. Finely chopped onion mixed with salt can also be used to treat warts. Use the juice and rub it on the warts three times a day.
9. Extracts from grapefruit seeds can also be used to treat warts. Cover the extract with plaster or band aid and in a month's time, the warts will disappear.

Try these effective methods at home to remove the warts, moles, and skin tags. These are inexpensive methods and the materials can be found mostly at home. You don't have to buy them because you can find them in your kitchen. To ensure maximum effectiveness, you must follow the directions on how to apply them properly.

By applying the remedies religiously, the unwanted moles, warts, and skin tags will disappear. The remedies require some time before results can be visibly seen but you mustn't lose hope. Keep applying the remedies and soon the skin lesions will disappear.

As you can see, using the home remedies can take months before the skin lesions disappear. For individuals who want to get rid of the skin lesions the fast way, the surgical methods are the best but you must prepare some money. So which method are you going to choose – the less expensive home remedies or the expensive surgical methods.

WARTS

Worried about irritating warts? There are a lot of ways on how to remove these irritating attachments from your skin. There are remedies that can be of big help and it's not even close with the idea of removing it through surgical treatments, scraping it off with a knife or even applying acidic compounds just to rid of it. Causes of these are because of infection made by viruses that can produce small mass in different parts of your skin and even under the soles of your feet.

Here are simple remedies on how to remove annoying skin infections.

Remedy # 1

If you have a wart, no matter where it is located, soak it in warm water about 15 to 25 minutes and towel dry. Soaking effects using warm water is used in order to moisten and make the wart tender so that the next steps will be more effective than the hardened wart. When the soaked wart has been all dried up, apply vinegar preferably apple cider using a cotton ball on the wart then leave it for about 15 minutes. Wash off the vinegar applied with clean water then dry it.

Remedy # 2

Get an aspirin then dissolve it with small drops of water then apply the solution on the wart. After applying the aspirin solution, cover the area with Band-Aid. You can do this procedure at least twice a day most likely upon waking up and before going to bed.

Remedy # 3

Using baking soda that is dissolve in water, rub the mixed solution to the wart at least three to four times every day. You can also use gauze that is soaked with the mixture of castor oil and baking soda then apply it on the wart. For it to be secured from dirt and dust or any foreign body that may be the cause of infectivity, put a Band-Aid on the area then leave it for the night.

Remedy # 4

In order to get rid of ugly plantar warts, you can do it naturally by applying the pulp of a ripe or even a raw banana peel on the wart then, to avoid being in contact with any untoward foreign substance, cover it with a clean cloth or Band-Aid. Remove the application only when you are going to take a bath. Do the procedure daily for a couple of months and observe how far it has changed.

For warts that are years old, the best suggestion is by applying chewed cashew on the wart. Do this for a couple of days. You'll notice that the wart is disappearing for about three to four weeks.

Remedy # 6

A dandelion stem can also be helpful in getting rid of warts. Rub the stem on the wart for two to three times every day until the wart is completely gone which is for about three to four weeks.

Remedy # 7

Crushed garlic is also an effective remedy that can be rubbed on the wart three times a day until complete disappearance of the wart, still for about three weeks to one month. Mashing a garlic glove so that it becomes moist and pulpy can also be put on the area. You will notice that the wart starts to gradually vanish a night after.

These procedures are only few tips on how to effectively do away with the warts.

ACNE

As a sufferer of acne, I was finally glad to get my life back after using a simple home remedy for acne that worked and got rid of my acne. I always hated life, I would awake in the morning and just couldn't face the mirror in my room, the sight of my own face would turn me off even more, I would just sit there feeling depressed.

No one can imagine the many different acne treatment solutions I tried, one after the other; it seemed as if nothing worked. But, I just never gave up hope that one day I would finally be able to rid myself of acne.

I would face the day asking myself one question: Is there an acne cure that works for me? I began to get depressed and tried to avoid my friends and family, my bedroom became my world, just living compound to those four walls. I used to spend hours and come up with very lame excuses, just to not face anyone.

The one day it happened, I saw an online ad that stated that an overlooked yet simple home remedy for acne can rid you of acne.

I read that page at least one hundred times, and decided to take a chance and see if this would work, and I am glad I did. Yes, it really worked, that simple home remedy for acne cured my acne. I was finally free.

That is where I also learned that many people believe they have acne, but they are actually only suffering from skin conditions that are related to acne, by simply balancing the skin PH value you can heal that condition. It is very important to understand what causes your acne, because only then can you discover a cure to rid yourself of that skin disease.

Nothing can change the way I feel now, because I have had many years of hiding and not being able to look anyone in the face, but there is hope for all, take a chance, and see if this simple home remedy for acne can be the answer to your problems.

Another problem I hear people talking about is that adult acne isn't as serious as teenage acne; well that is a whole load of hog wash. Acne is horrible no matter at what age, I guess those touting that rumor has never suffered with acne, and they have no clue what they are talking about.

I can only offer you hope and insist you never give up trying to find your acne cure, as each one of us is different, but we seek the same gold and that is to find a simple home remedy for acne that will not cost too much.

My best friend face was constantly red, he thought he had acne, well he didn't and that is where the problem starts, just because you think its acne, that doesn't mean it is.

Get the facts, and learn the exact steps I took to cure my acne by following this simple home remedy for acne. I know my English isn't the best and I am no doctor, but I do know what worked for me.

Green Tea - A Natural Remedy For Acne

Natural remedies have become very popular in recent years. People have stopped looking at the expensive medications and creams to cure various conditions, and have started looking at remedies found closer to home. This is, in part, because they are less expensive, but they are also on hand and easily obtained.

Acne is a common condition in teens and adults alike, and is no exception to the theory that a home remedy can sometimes be better. If it's worked for many years, why wouldn't it work now? One such remedy believed to aid in the healing of acne is green tea.

While many teas are fermented, green tea instead, is steamed soon after being picked so as to prevent the oxidation of its leaves. This helps to retain the active substances the leaves contain. Camellia Sinensis, or as we know it, green tea extract, contains a high content of Polyphenol, along with other important antioxidants.

Green tea can serve many purposes, and it is recommended for a number of reasons. It acts as an anti-bacterial substance, decreasing hormonal activity. Since acne is often caused by hormones, which produce excess oil and clog pores, thereby causing blemishes, green tea could be a good remedy for this problem.

The antioxidants contained in green tea have been shown as very beneficial to acne prevention because they help the body fight against free radicals that cause cell and tissue damage. Green tea also has very few potential side effects, especially when compared to other acne products and medications.

Because of its advantages, green tea is also used in various creams and other topical products used to treat acne. When compared with other commonly used acne treatments, it ranked high, because of its natural anti-bacterial properties. Other products containing green tea extract are also sold and developed, and are available as herbal remedies. It can be purchased as a cream.

Green Tea and honeysuckle is often called "Pimple Tea" in China. It also helps your body rid itself of toxins, which helps prevent acne. Green tea is also easily available. It can be purchased in most stores that carry various herbal and other natural remedies, and can also be bought through many on-line sources. It comes in the form of tea that you drink, or can be purchased in the form of the cream mentioned above.

Drinking green tea will help cleanse your body from the inside out, while applying the topical cream, which goes directly onto the skin, will help cure and prevent acne at the source. No matter how you choose to use it, it can serve many purposes, and may be a welcome alternative to harsh products or unwanted medications.

Chapter 2- Remedies for Aches and Pains

ARTHRITIS

People generally think of arthritis as an 'old persons' disease. In reality anyone can be afflicted with this painful condition. In order to alleviate the pain associated with this disease, many people have turned to prescription or over the counter remedies. Unfortunately, the side effects from these remedies were often as bad as the pain from the arthritis itself. That may be why so many people are turning safer, gentler arthritis home remedies.

While you should never just stop taking a prescription your doctor has given you without talking to him first, you may be able to combine both home remedies along with your prescription which may make it possible to cut back on the amount of pain relievers you have to take thus diminishing many of the negative side effects. Always talk to your doctor first.

Something as simple as using a heating pad when you are sitting at your computer or watching TV. might offer you a lot of relief for your swollen and achy joints. Also make sure you keep your home comfortably heated during the winter months so you don't get cold.

Many people have reported that having a nice long soak in a warm bath has helped them find some pain relief too. Another benefit is that this can help relax you which is something very precious when you are living with such a painful condition.

Another tip that may help is to use warm olive oil and massage it into your sore joints. No need to stop at just your joints either, massage the tendons leading to your joints. For example, if your knees are sore, massage a little up your thighs too.

While it may not smell that great, many people have reported getting relief by massaging with warm vinegar. This may be a great thing to try when the in laws come for a visit!

The general rule of thumb is to apply ice before the joints are swollen. If they are already inflamed you should only apply heat. If you get to them before they are swollen ice can work very effectively. Generally if any treatment hurts you should stop.

Using a cream or ointment specifically created to ease joint pain can help provide relief overnight. Apply the cream at bedtime and you may have a less painful time sleeping, which means you'll actually be rested the next day.

As difficult as it may be to do, most doctors recommend that you try to stay active. The more you work your joints the looser you'll be able to keep them. Try low impact activities such as yoga or swimming. These exercises are a great way to stay in shape and keep your joints limber and they won't stress your joints further since they have virtually no impact on you.

You don't have to suffer or rely solely on prescription or over the counter arthritis pain relief. There are many simple, yet highly effective arthritis home remedies. As with anything, some will work better for some people than others so it's really just a matter of finding the best combination of treatments for you.

BACK PAIN

Majority of people often experience back pain at some point in their lives. The reason may be vague and there are cases that the causes are undefined. However, some experts would agree that one of the typical causes of back pain is muscle imbalance.

Throughout the day, most Americans would only spend time sitting and not moving. And frequently, the activities we perform often lead us to the couch and the desks. That's all there is to it. And so to add mobility to our bodies, we go to the gyms and make the imbalance even more severe.

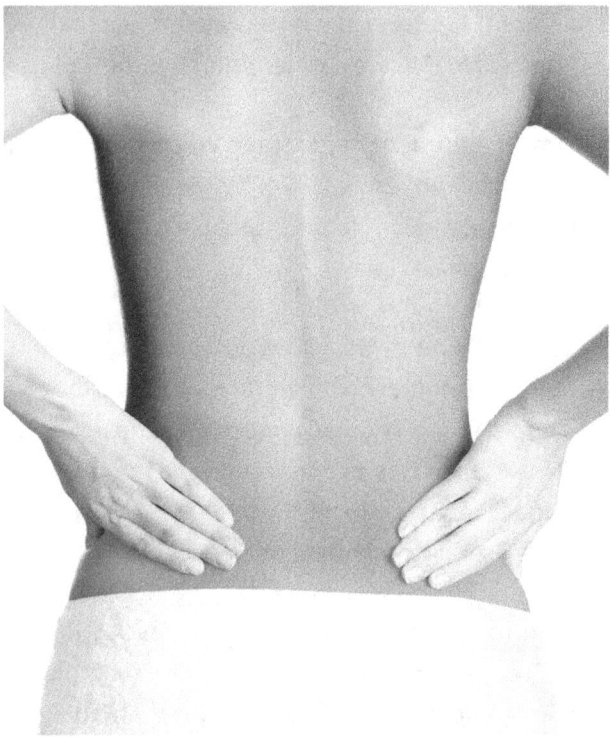

The first step to back pain remedy is to identify the muscle imbalance in our body. These pull our bones, joints and spine in some places out of their natural locations. Then stretch the tight and often not used muscles to strengthen to reinstate strength.

It is normally not easy to identify what trigger muscle imbalances. But with some basic knowledge on how the body system works, it may well be easier to observe which muscles are better used than others and where the body typically hurts.

Or you may choose to use other methods other than focusing on the imbalances of the muscles without going too far from exercising. One such option is the yoga. In opposition with the first back pain remedy we discussed, yoga needs to be thoroughly understood. One needs to have a good foundation on the background of this art and how does it work. And restrictions must be carefully observed.

There is a host of methods for treating back pain, ranging from conventional methods and alternative therapies. Whatever way one wants it to be, the result may always be affected by psychological expectations and beliefs on the outcome. Say in acupuncture, doctors may claim that it works for some and not for others. How is this; probably because people believe in the effects of the said method but may not actually be the case for all. We are not raising arguments on this issue; we are just presenting what is factual. Nor are we proving that contemporary medicine works more efficiently than that of the more traditional methods. Anything that works well for the patients will continue on working well; unless other factors impede it.

The thing is it really doesn't matter what back pain remedy we use, we only have to seek for what is effective and which of them creates more productive results. In this, it might be true that the end justifies the means.

HEADACHES

Everybody has definitely experienced a headache once in his or her lifetime. Since it is one of the indispensable and common illnesses everyone experiences, people have learned to find ways to relieve the discomfort brought by headache.

Headaches are usually caused by physical and emotional stress. If you are dying to find a solution to your persistent headache, try taking in over the counter remedies like aspirin, acetaminophen, and ibuprofen. But if you are not a big fan of prescribed or over the counter medications, try these home remedies for a change.

1. Try using compresses or cold packs. For tension headaches— the most common form of headache—try applying a warm or cold compress to your forehead and the base of your neck to numb the pain.
2. Try using heat. If cold compresses wouldn't work out for you, try using a warm washcloth or a hot water bottle can ease pain.
3. Develop a routine of deep breathing exercises. If you suffer from headaches very often, try sitting in a darkened room, take in deep breaths using your nose, and let it pass through your mouth.
4. Experience the wonders of acupressure. By squeezing the web of skin between and the thumb through acupressure, it can reduce the pains and can help you relax.
5. Try relaxation techniques such as meditation, yoga, and biofeedback. By trying these relaxation techniques, the person who suffers from headache can feel the pain flowing out of the head. It can also help reduce stress.
6. Relieve the affected area by applying ointment with heat. Ben-Gay or Icy Hot rubbed on forehead or on the base of the neck can give a soothing warm feeling to your head.
7. The power of music. Try listening to a relaxing music while lying down or resting.

8. Exercise regularly. Physical activities like regular exercise can relieve stress because it can loosen up the knots and balls of pain in your head.
9. Get enough sleep. Having six to eight hours of sleep can help you soothe your tired nerves. But, beware of sleeping more than 10 hours because it can cause major headache as well.
10. If possible, use a neck pillow in bed. If you are prone to experiencing morning headaches, try using a neck pillow to your neck while you sleep.
11. Totally eliminate caffeine, salt, MSG, and chocolate in your diet. Load up on lots of fruits, veggies, and water to keep your body well hydrated. - If you can, avoid bright light because it leads to a major headache once your squint.
12. Don't skip meals. Skipping meals can lead to low blood sugar. When your sugar level goes down, your blood vessels in the brain tightens that leads to headache.
13. Don't eat foods that have nitrates, sulfites, and MSG because these are primary headache causers. Also avoid aged cheeses and nuts so you won't experience headaches.
14. Don't smoke and avoid smoke-filled rooms.

TOOTHACHES

Emergency home remedies for toothaches are always going to be searched for, simply because of the nature of many toothaches. They have a tendency to erupt at night when the person is sound asleep and the chance of immediately visiting a dentist is not possible.

What you can do in a toothache emergency will depend on what is causing the problem. First of all check that there is no food stuck in between the teeth or in any open cavities. A simple brushing and flossing in this instance is often enough to bring ease.

Toothaches can also be as a result of a sensitivity to hot or cold drinks and foods. If this is the case then a home remedies for toothaches that will work involves the reduction or elimination of these foods from the diet. Sensitivity to foods and drinks could also be an indication that there may be some further damage to the tooth or gums and at the earliest convenience a checkup at the dentist should be arranged.

If there is decay involved in the toothache, then the home remedies for toothaches that are then applicable involve bringing relief from the pain and not in curing the toothache. Putting ice on the painful tooth is a good way to numb the nerve and reduce any inflammation that may be present. This will give the sufferer some well needed pain free time as they wait to see their dentist.

Make sure that if you can at all stand it that the teeth are brushed and cleaned thoroughly. This will not only remove food, but it will also remove bacteria that can be hanging around and causing the pain in your tooth. Cleaning the teeth is probably the last thing on the mind of someone who is suffering the rage of a toothache, but the solution to your problem could well be a simple cleaning of the teeth.

If you have a toothache emergency when you are out on a windy day, it could be an indication that the wind is getting into a hole that's in one of your teeth! This might sound odd, but it's true, some people find out that all is not well within their mouths by feeling pain when they are out and about. In this case one of the home remedies for toothaches that will work until you can get to your dentist is to simply keep your mouth closed.

Nothing will beat staving off a toothache, like brushing your teeth at least twice a day; in doing this, you head off many of the complications that can lead to a toothache. So brush twice a day and chances are you'll avoid that toothache emergency!

NATURAL TOOTHACHE REMEDIES

Not many people are aware of the fact that several herbs can be used in the relief of toothache pain. Natural herbs such as cloves, calendula, tarragon, and yarrow can be used to help relieve the pain until you can get to the dentist. For many years, different cultures have counted on herbs to help get the pain of a toothache control and get temporary relief.

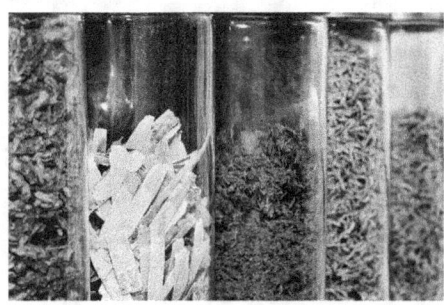

Native Americans for example, used the inner bark found in the butternut tree to their gums to get relief from toothaches. The butternut tree is found in North America, and is also the cousin of the black walnut tree. Butternut trees are found along rivers in well-drained soil, rich woods, and even in back yards. Once the tree matures, it can reach heights of up to 60 feet, with the bark being light grey in color, and the leaves and the fruit resembling the black walnut tree. The bark of the tree can be applied to the gums, helping to alleviate toothache pain.

Yarrow on the other hand, can be found in Asia, Europe, and North America. It normally grows wild in meadows, fields, and in open wood lands. The root of yarrow is what contains the anesthetic effect. If you apply the fresh root of yarrow to your tooth or gums, it will help to stop the pain - until you can get an appointment with the dentist and get it taken care of.

The herb known as clove is an evergreen tree, native to tropical areas. These days however, it can be found throughout the world. As many already know, the dried flower bud of clove is what contains the medicine. The oil from clove, when used on a toothache, will help to stop the pain almost immediately. If you compare cloves to other natural toothache remedies, you'll find clove to be the best.

For many years, natural herbs have been used to stop toothache pain. Hundreds of years ago, herbs were the only way to stop the pain. Dentists were just starting to come around, although they didn't have near the equipment and sophistication that they have these days. Even though teeth were pulled during these times, it normally happened with alcohol to numb the pain then pliers to remove the tooth.

Throughout the course of time, herbs have proven to be very effective with stopping toothache pain. If you are interested in herbs or have any questions about them, you shouldn't hesitate to ask your dentist his opinion. Dentists know herbs, and should be able to recommend natural remedies to you if you request them. The next time you experience the pain of a toothache - you should always remember that herbs are a great way to relieve the pain.

EARACHES

Earache is one of those things that often first occur when we are babies, continues on and off throughout childhood and even has occasions to occur as adults. Home remedies for earache then can be useful bits of information to have at your disposal to counter this often painful condition.

Often usually occurring when there is a cold or flu or sinus problems, earaches are often the result of the tube between the throat and the middle ear being infected and becoming blocked.

Because of its antibacterial and antiviral properties, garlic is a great home remedy ingredient that helps in a variety of conditions, aches and pains. Not surprising then that it has its place and uses as one of the home remedies for earache. The simplest way is to eat a couple of cloves of raw garlic per day as this will help to kill off the bacteria in the ear canal. Garlic can also be used as an ear drop, dropped into the ear. However, using concentrated garlic in this way should be avoided because it will irritate the inner ear. What should be mixed with the garlic is an oil called mullein.

Mixing up a massage oil of lavender, tea tree and chamomile and then massaging the outer ear with this oil has been known to offer relief to earaches. It can also be applied to the ear itself by dipping a piece of cotton into the oil and then placing it in the ear.

The use of warm olive oil dropped into the ear has been used as a good home remedy for earaches. All that is required is for the oil to be warmed slightly and then a few drops, dropped into the ear. This keeps the ear lubricated and helps with any irritation within the ear.

Some particularly good home remedies for earache involve what can be done to stop an earache occurring in the first place. Often times a plane journey can trigger an earache. This is because of the changes in pressure as the plane lands and takes off. We are often told to swallow at this point in the journey and for good reason. Swallowing helps to equalize the pressure within the ear and the atmosphere we're in. Further flying tips that will help to equalize pressure in the ear and the environment include the sucking on candy, keeping the mouth moving and stretching and swallowing as deeply as you possible.

Above all, avoid poking around in the ear and placing foreign objects in the ear. The ear is a delicate and important organ and should be looked after and cared for with this in mind.

Chapter 3- Remedies for Ear Infections

Ear infections are a fairly common occurrence for many people. The ear canals are very prone to developing bacterial and fungal infections, especially in young children. In fact, each year over 20 million doctor's visits are related to ear infections in children alone.

If you're a parent, or even an adult who gets frequent ear infections, then you may want to find some information about ear infection and remedy. Keep on reading to learn about the causes, symptoms and ways to treat an ear infection.

Ear infection is otherwise known as otitis media. It is an infection which takes place right behind an ear drum. It is often caused by bacteria that come from an outside source, but simple water can also turn an ear canal into a breeding ground for infection.

Infecting bacteria usually come through a channel called the Eustachian tube, which connects the back of the threat to the inner ear. When it comes to ear infection and curing it, it's important to understand how this works.

Normally this tube provides a way to drain the fluids that get built up as part of the ear's normal workings. When there's a problem with this tube, ear infections occur. One way this can happen is through other diseases. For example, the common cold can damage some of the tiny hair follicles in this tube, causing them to stop working properly. This leads to bacteria buildup and eventually ear infection.

The next thing to understand about ear infection and its cures are the symptoms. The most common symptom of ear infection is simply pain. The pain of an ear infection can vary from being mildly annoying to extremely painful. In some cases, there may also be some kind of discharge that comes from the ear. If the infection spreads, it can lead to a number of other symptoms, including flu-like symptoms such as fever and vomiting. In some cases, it can put a person off balance and cause dizziness.

When it comes to ear infection and remedy, there are a number of options for relieving and curing the problem. Most doctors will prescribe a prescription antibiotic that will help give your body a boost in fighting off the infection.

However, most people dealing with an ear infection need relief right away, and visiting a doctor may not be possible for hours or even days. In those cases, there are many home remedies that can be used to help deal with ear infections. Sometimes, simple over the counter ear drops can be enough to combat the pain and irritation of ear infection. If that doesn't work, there are many more outlandish home remedies. You can use a number of different items that you may have around your home to help get ear infection relief.

Some examples include vinegar, lemon juice, and even garlic cooked in oil. You may need to test out some different home remedies to find one that works for you. However, before trying any home remedies it's a good idea to visit a doctor at least once.

HOME REMEDY FOR AN EAR INFECTION

A home remedy for an ear infection may be your best option if you are a parent. Children tend to get ear infections often and it can be costly going to the doctor each time. It's especially bothersome when you are on vacation and you need a quick fix. Luckily there are many treatments you can do yourself. However, before trying any home remedies it's a good idea to visit a doctor at least once.

People have been dealing with ear infections using the products they have sitting in their home for many years. These are things that have been working since the days when doctors weren't readily available, so people had to treat themselves. You can take advantage of these treatments too.

A hot compress is a good option for at home or on the go. Have the child hold the hot compress to their ear with a towel or washcloth wrapped around it. You will also want them to lie on the side that is infected. This will force the build-up to come out of the ear while helping with the pain.

You probably have a bottle of hydrogen peroxide in your home and you can use this as a method of treating an ear infection. All you need is a couple drops into the infected ear and let it drop down in. The hydrogen peroxide will kill the infection.

Lemon juice can have a similar effect to hydrogen peroxide if you have that in your home and want to use something more natural. Lemon juice is an acidic which will neutralize the base chemical properties of the bacteria, stopping the infection.

Garlic and onions combined with olive oil can create an all-natural solution to an ear infection. You'll need to simmer those ingredients together with a small amount of water. When it cools, use an eyedropper to put a few drops into the infected ear. Let it soak, and within 24 hours the infection will be gone.

Vinegar is found in most homes, and if you have it too you can use that to create an ear infection fighting solution. A combination of 50 percent vinegar and 50 percent water will make a powerful cleaning solution that is safe for anyone's ear.

Although it is a strange use for a liquor, vodka can also cure an ear infection, and not by drinking it. Dab a small amount of vodka onto a cotton ball and press it against the infected ear. Make sure some of the vodka drips into the ear. The strong alcohol content will remove the infection without causing harm like a pure alcohol would.

You can choose any of these home remedies and see which one works best for your children. Once you find one you like, you can continue to use that home remedy for an ear infection each time they get one. Be sure and remember that home remedies may not work and if the infections or pain continue, you should consult with your professional health care provider.

Chapter 4- Remedies for Hypertension

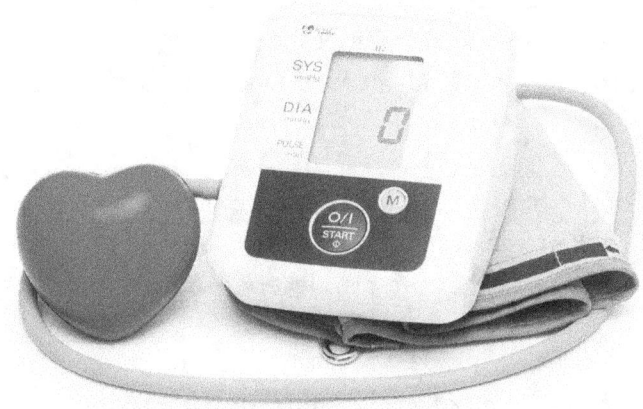

Over one third of Americans have hypertension. All those people think they need to be put on meds to get their blood pressure back to normal. For some people that is the only way to get their blood pressure into normal ranges. However, for others, there are natural remedies for lowering blood pressure.

One of the best ways if not the best way, is exercise. Exercise is a wonderful remedy for a huge number of ailments. For people that are overweight, have high cholesterol, and high blood pressure.

You don't have to hit the gym 7 days a week, or workout so hard you almost pass out. All it takes is a brisk walk for 20 to 30 minutes a day. That's all you have to do is just get your heart pumping and you are on your way.

Another remedy is cutting out fatty foods. Try to stop eating at fast food restaurants; those are the worst places to go if you are trying to get healthy. There have been documentaries about what fast food can do to your body and your blood pressure.

Cut salt out of your diet all together. There are other things out there to add flavor to your food. Stop eating fried food, fried chicken, fried pork chops, fried fish; it's all bad for you. If you still want to eat those kinds of food, well, you can. Just bake, broil or grill it.

One of the hardest things I had to do is cut back on my sodas. It's true, look on the back of the labels of the next drink you have. You would be amazed at the high level of sodium that goes into each serving.

I know the alternative for soda doesn't sound too appealing; however water is the best alternative for you. Water doesn't do the damage that soda does and it's a heck of a lot cheaper. It will make a world of difference in the way you feel as well.

Eat plenty of fruit people, apples, grapes you name it, it's good for you. Try to eat grapes for a snack instead of pigging out with candy and potato chips. They taste just as good and it's a whole lot cheaper and better for you.

I know all these remedies may be tougher to do then I make it out to be. However you have to take that first step. I wouldn't recommend trying to cut everything out all at one time. I would take one step one week, then another in a couple of weeks and so on and so on.

It's your life people, and you are the only one that can determine if you want to do this. If you decide to go with these hypertension natural remedies, your body will thank you for it, and so will the people who love you.

NATURAL REMEDIES FOR HIGH BLOOD PRESSURE

Most people know that having high blood pressure can lead to very serious medical issues. We all know that high blood pressure, if left untreated, can lead to heart disease, stroke, and kidney problems. The bad thing is that there are a lot of things we don't know about high blood pressure, such as what causes it. Also a lot of the prescription drugs prescribed for high blood pressure have dangerous side effects. If you want to get your blood pressure under control, try these high blood pressure home remedies.

It is estimated that upwards of 95% of the people who have high blood pressure don't even know that they are at risk. That is why high blood pressure is often referred to as the silent killer. There are a lot of things you can do that can help you lower your high blood pressure.

Of course, if you are under a doctor's care and taking prescription medications, talk to your doctor before you make any changes. Even though these home remedies are all natural, that doesn't mean that you still can't have a potentially dangerous interaction with your other medications.

Here are some things you can try:

1. Use fresh lemon juice, about half a lemon, and add to an 8 ounce glass of water. Drink throughout your day, two to three hours apart.
2. Mix a tablespoon full of gooseberry juice with some honey and drink every day in the morning. Gooseberry helps to keep your blood flowing smoothly.

3. Take 1 tsp. of fenugreek seeds and add to a cup of water and drink daily in the morning and at night before bed. Doing this for about 25 days can help lower your high blood pressure.

4. Eating fresh papaya daily, on an empty stomach, has been shown in some people to help lower blood pressure.

5. And last, but not least, garlic. This may be one of the best known remedies for treating high blood pressure. Most people recommend taking about 1 clove a day and have noticed a significant decrease in their blood pressure in about 3 months. You can easily add it to many of the foods you prepare.

6. Exercise, particularly those, such as yoga, that are relaxing can help lower your blood pressure. The more you exercise the healthier your body will become and depending on the cause of your high blood pressure this could help lower your high blood pressure by giving you some much needed relaxation techniques.

If you are obese the exercises will provide the added benefit of helping you lose weight which will not only help with the high blood pressure but which can also help clear up, or prevent, many other health related issues.

Don't allow high blood pressure to put your health at risk. With so many potential side effects, you want to make sure you get, and keep, your high blood pressure under control, and you don't need to solely rely on expensive prescription drugs and all the side effects they come with. Use these simple high blood pressure home remedies to get this dangerous disease under control once and for all.

CHAPTER 5- REMEDIES FOR HEARTBURN AND INDIGESTION

It's good to know that many home remedies for heartburn are often based around foods that are readily available in many kitchens. However, understanding just what is going on when heartburn hits will often help to minimize and cure heartburn in itself.

Heartburn happens when the strong acid in the stomach, that is used to digest and break down the foods we eat, finds its way up the esophagus (food tube). It is this acid that burns the lining of the esophagus, causing the familiar and unpleasant sensation of burning. There is a muscle that is supposed to keep the acid in the stomach where it belongs, but if for whatever reason this muscle malfunctions, then it leaves the way open for the acid to escape into the esophagus.

One of the most common home remedies for heartburn has to be the eating of soda crackers. The soda cracker remedy has been handed down through the generations for one reason, it works! As long as the crackers are salt free, since salt increases the sodium in the body, which further influences the amount of acidity in your stomach, soda crackers are a convenient and useful snack that aids digestion. The crackers contain bio-carbonate soda which works by lessening the acid. Incidentally, for the same reasons, a mixture of water and baking soda is also a quick and simple aid to digestion.

Some sufferers with heartburn also swear by eating a handful of blanched almonds. This works because almonds have properties that neutralize the symptoms of heartburn and calm the unpleasant burning sensation. What also works in exactly the same way as almonds is eating boiled plain brown rice. Not only that, but plain brown rice is also one of those home remedies for heartburn that falls into the category of foods that are 'easy and simple to digest'. Any foods that are easy and simple to digest will often help diminish the risk of heartburn because not so many digestive juices and acid is needed to break down these foods.

The other home remedies for heartburn that are often used, are centered around the avoidance of practices that will encourage the acid from the stomach finding its way into the esophagus. These remedies start by doing some obvious things like not eating too close to bedtime and so give the body time to fully digest the foods that have been eaten before retiring. Also simply elevating the head when asleep is another remedy that can be successfully used. Sleeping in this position will naturally help gravity keep the acid down in the stomach where it belongs.

A general rule of thumb where heartburn is concerned is to keep an eye on your diet and remain at a healthy weight. Drink plenty of water between meals, rather than during meals, which can lead to the stomach over filling and so encourage the escape of the acid back up the food tube.

Simple and straightforward solutions to managing and stopping heartburn!

Soothe Nighttime Heartburn And Indigestion

Who hasn't bolted upright in the night, awakened by a sudden and terrible burning sensation in the pit of their stomach? Whether you indulged in some overly spicy chili, or overdid it on those late-night leftovers, these quick heartburn remedies will soothe your fiery stomach and help you get back to sleep!

Mihalis Kapakolis

1. The first thing you'll want to do when you're awakened by heartburn pain is to stand up. This helps keep the acid at bay while you go and get a full glass of cool water.

2. Drink the whole glass of water, and follow it with a mixture of 1 tablespoon of baking soda, and half a glass of water. Be careful though, if you have high blood pressure or are pregnant, this can cause water retention or increase your blood pressure.

3. DON'T drink milk or suck on mints to relieve heartburn. Milk might feel nice and cool going down, but it actually contains fats and proteins that cause your stomach to secrete MORE acid and make your heartburn worse! Mints, while they may feel soothing, actually relax the small valve between your esophagus and stomach, whose purpose it is to actually KEEP acid at bay! When this valve is relaxed, more acid can seep up and aggravate heartburn symptoms!

4. This is going to sound strange, but downing a teaspoon of vinegar can help soothe heartburn immediately! Why give your stomach MORE acid when it already seems to have enough, you ask? Sometimes, heartburn is caused as a result of too little acid, and vinegar helps quell indigestion by giving your stomach a little extra "juice" (no pun intended!) to do its job!

5. Certain foods can cause nighttime heartburn, including: soda pop or beverages with caffeine (which you shouldn't be drinking before bed anyway!), alcohol, garlic, chocolate (sorry!), citrus fruits, tomatoes and tomato-based products. Avoiding these types of food can help ease your indigestion if you frequently find yourself awakened with that intolerable burning!

6. Eating a banana each day works like an antacid to soothe heartburn. If you're already stricken with indigestion, eating pineapple or papaya (or drinking the juice) can help settle your stomach naturally. Some people also claim that eating a teaspoon of mustard (yuck!) can work immediately.

7. Avoid eating at least two hours before you go to sleep. Those late night snacks can keep your stomach busy all night and prevent you from easing into a deep, restful sleep. You may also find that sleeping on your left side or sleeping at a somewhat upright angle can keep acid down where it belongs.

If you are awakened by heartburn on a regular basis or the pain is severe, or if you have heartburn with vomiting, you'll want to consult your doctor immediately as it may be a sign of a more serious condition such as an ulcer. Above all, avoid spicy, fatty and caffeine-containing foods before bed, and you should be able to drift off to sleep easily.

CHAPTER 6- REMEDIES FOR ORAL CONDITIONS

CANKER SORES

If you have canker sores you will definitely be looking around for effective canker sore remedies. Canker sores can be very painful and may be triggered by certain foods, stress, or injury to the inside of your mouth.

Foods that are acidic and can trigger a canker sore are foods like lemons, oranges, pineapples, figs, apples, tomatoes or strawberries. Other causes may be dental problems like a sharp tooth or ill-fitting dentures. Sometimes the friction from braces can cause an outbreak, also. Acidic juices and carbonated drinks can also contribute to the formation or exacerbation of canker sores.

There are two types of canker sores, simple and complex. Simple canker sores are caused by the foods or dental problems discussed above. Complex canker sores are usually caused by some underlying medical condition that causes immune system depletion like Celiac disease or Crohn's. Vitamin and mineral deficiencies play a major role in the development of canker sores.

Some people may think that canker sores and cold sores are one and the same. This is not true. Cold sores are caused by a virus and develop on the outside of the mouth. Canker sores develop on the inside of the mouth. Though canker sores and cold sores can be equally as painful, they are not the same thing and both require different treatment.

If you have a painful sore or sores in your mouth, feel a burning sensation or rough spot develop before the sores appear, have a low grade fever, swollen lymph glands or feel sluggish, you may be fairly certain you have canker sores.

When you have an active canker sore you will need to steer clear of the types of foods we discussed earlier because they will not only cause you pain when you eat them but they may even make your condition worse.

If the sores do not start to heal on their own in a few days or you cannot eat or drink, you should not hesitate to see your dentist to receive canker sore remedies. You will also want to do yourself a favor and get a toothbrush with a soft bristle. Keeping your mouth clean is a good way to help the canker sores heal up quicker.

Some other symptoms that should prompt you to see your dentist are unusually large sores, sores that spread, sores that last more than three weeks, sores that cause severe pain, or you have a high fever.

There is no cure and canker sores can happen to anyone but with care and learning to avoid certain acidic or even spicy foods you may be able to reduce their frequency and severity. If the pain is too severe your doctor or dentist should be willing to prescribe you with a pain med that is effective in reducing the amount of pain you are feeling.

Over the counter canker sore remedies are available and may help with the healing of your canker sores. Over the counter pain medications may also help so you won't need to ask for a prescription from your doctor or dentist.

COLD SORES

Having a cold sore can make you uncomfortable and just generally irritated and unhappy. While there is no cure for cold sores, there are some cold sore home remedy treatments that many people have gotten relief with. You may or may not experience the same results but it's worth a try to alleviate some of the pain and discomfort you're feelings, isn't it?

Cold sores are caused by the herpes simplex 1 virus. This is not the same virus that causes genital herpes which is herpes simplex 2. The simplex virus 1 can be dormant in your body, often since childhood, until the right set of triggers occur and trigger a full-fledged outbreak.

Of course if you can identify what triggers your outbreak you may be able to stop some of the outbreaks even before they start. Simple things like making sure you eat nutritiously (I know you may be wondering what that has to do with anything but the healthier your body is in general the easier time it will have fighting off all types of illnesses and infections).

Go easy on the things that aren't good for you like nicotine, too much caffeine and junk food. Instead get enough sleep, keep your body hydrated and try to keep your stress levels at a reasonable level. If you have a high stress job, for example, try to at least learn some techniques for de-stressing a little bit.

You could take a yoga class, learn to meditate or just go kick boxing, whatever you can do that will help you stay calm.

Now, here are some cold sore home remedy treatments for you to try;

1. Take an ice cube and apply it directly to the cold sore. Hold it in place until the cube has melted. This can be a little

uncomfortable but if you can get rid of the cold sore more quickly it might be worth it. Once the ice cube has melted take a dry towel and carefully dry the cold sore. Dab it, don't rub it. Once it's dry take a little rubbing alcohol on a cotton ball and dab the cold sore. This will sting, but the cold sore will be a little bit numb from the ice so not as bad as it could.

2. Take Lysine when you first feel a little tingle on your lip (this is usually the first sign that you are getting a cold sore) Use it 3 times daily and hopefully this will prevent the cold sore from actually forming in the first place. If you've never heard of Lysine, just go down to your local drug store and ask them where to find it.

3. Don't re-infect yourself by using the same toothbrush or toothpaste. Buy a new toothbrush and toothpaste at the first sign of an outbreak.

When you have an outbreak, or to prevent an outbreak, use one or more simple cold sore home remedy treatments to find the relief you need much more quickly than you might have thought possible.

BAD BREATH

Bad breath or halitosis is probably the most shameful oral condition a person may have. This dental condition will even alter your professional life, even your very personal being. It is therefore important to have it treated as soon as you discover that you have it in your mouth. And if you really feel bad in unveiling this very intimate hygienic condition, you can simply go for the bad breath home remedy formulated for those that have it but not willing to share it even to oral professionals. But before the treatment, you have to ensure that you really have it by doing the following revealing tips:

1. Prove to yourself that you really have bad breath to prevent from overreacting or overdoing your oral hygiene. Lick your wrist and have it dried in about five seconds. Then smell it. How does it smell to you? How it smells is just the same as how your breath smells to other people.

2. If you have a bad breath, it is now time to know how bad it is. Get a metal or silver spoon and scrape the back part of your tongue. By the way, that part of your tongue is the posterior and the front part is the anterior. The posterior is where the halitosis bacteria thrive. Smell the residue that is left into the spoon after scraping. How does it smell to you this time? If it is worse than you think, too bad, you have a chronic bad breath!

Now that you know what level of bad breath you will be dealing with, here is a list of useful home remedies you can use to treat yourself in the comfort of your home:

1. Improving your oral hygienic method. This time, it's not enough for you to toothbrush alone; you also need to use mouthwash and deodorizer. Do this regularly and properly.

2. You also have to brush your tongue, starting on the back and going outwards.

3. When you eat dairy foods, meats, and fish, make sure you brush your teeth. Or at least, gargle mouthwash if a toothbrush is not available.

4. Drink a lot of fluids with the exemption of coffee and alcohol as these beverages can even aggravate your oral condition.

5. Eat fibrous foods. These types of foods are very safe for your oral condition.

6. Have your breath tested on your kids or nieces and nephews. They will surely not mind after all by being creative on how to do it. One of the most effective ways is by making fun of it or just comparing your smells. Or if

even kids make you think you will look a fool in testing your breath odor, you can use the above mentioned procedures to track your improvement.

If you are satisfied with how you are doing, don't be settled and go back to your slack oral hygiene practices. Continue practicing what you have already learned and you will surely be more than happy to know that the chronic bad breath you once experience is totally gone. It will even be more satisfying to know that no one knew you went over it in the sanctuaries of your home.

Therefore, no one will even believe that you once have it because you never officially admitted it.

CHAPTER 7- REMEDIES FOR DEPRESSION AND STRESS

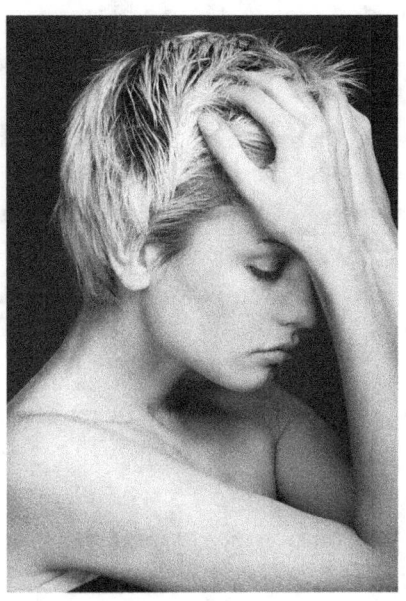

DEPRESSION

Depression home remedies may just be what you need if you want to shake the blues and your depression. The American bluesman, John Lee Hooker, spoke the truth when he said about the blues, "It's about being human, see? Everybody gets the blues. Even a rich man gets the blues sometime." No one is immune from it but everyone can beat it. Using some of these depression home remedies may help you get out of your depression before you need outside help and before it takes too much of a toll on you and your family.

Enjoy The Ride:

One of the depression home remedies that you may want to try is sitting back and enjoying the ride. This doesn't mean that being depressed is a good thing and something to enjoy, but it is a natural part of life. Life is many times like a roller coaster. Every once in a while you have dips in the ride. Take it for what it is, just a little low spot, and don't make it into a bigger deal than it really is.

Get Active:

Many times what makes a depressed situation worse is sitting around and pondering it. The more you dwell on it, the worse it may become. To get your mind off of it try doing something active to preoccupy you. Do something that takes you out of your house, out of your situation.

Go for a run or a walk. Go hit the gym or play some basketball. Go see a friend and play some checkers or cards. Go to the library and read a book that has nothing to do with what is going on now. It may seem ironic that one of the depression home remedies would be to get you out of the home but it will be effective none-the-less.

"It's Alright to Cry":

No one says that you have to let anyone see you do it but crying can be very therapeutic and cleansing. It can help you come to grips with whatever it is that has you depressed and is a good way to release what is building up inside. It doesn't matter how big you are or how tough you are, crying will help you and is one of the better depression home remedies.

Do Something Boring:

This may seem like an odd thing to tell someone to do, especially when one of the other depression home remedies was to get active. It can, however, be another great way to distract you. Find a spider web and study the patterns, following the lines. Count the tiles on your wall. Follow the grains of wood on the floor and look for patterns. Even get out some crayons or coloring pencils and draw or create patterns. This will help to settle your mind and may help you relax.

Use these methods soon after you first start feeling the blues or a bit depressed. If you have these feelings for more than two weeks, then you may need professional help. Before it gets to that point, though, try these depression home remedies and kick the blues out the door.

STRESS

There are numerous methods involved in the reduction of stress. For this article, I shall look at the simpler ones. Yoga, Tai Chi and sport may not be something you are accustomed to doing each day. Other than exercise and hitting the pharmaceutical cupboard, there are even simpler remedies to relieve stress. Here is a checklist of items to action each day.

1. 1.Early to bed, early to rise. The expression fits well into a balanced day though it's more about the controlled sleeping patterns. It's not a good thing to have only a few hours of sleep each night. Have a good night's sleep; 7 hours each night fits well into a stress relieving pattern.
2. 2.Don't drink vast amounts of caffeine as this disrupts your daily balance. If you are prone to drinking too much caffeine, try cutting down and fit some decaffeinated coffee and tea into your day. Yes, caffeine gives you a burst of energy to enable you to feel more alert but the effect is short.
3. 3.Eat lots of fruit, get the needed daily vitamins. Apples and bananas are very healthy supplements as part of your daily food intake. Bananas are not fattening and apples help the

immune system. Don't eat too much processed food; concentrate on drinking and eating the required vitamins.

4. 4.Salt raises your blood pressure, so keep an eye on salty foods being consumed. Higher blood pressure will contribute to your stress levels and is a killer.

5. 5.Look back over the past week at the positive aspects that made you feel good. Did something occur that attracted an experience of joy and laughter? Send some time focusing on that moment as it will allow you to attract good feelings into your mind and smother any negative impact from the day.

6. 6.If you must reach for pharmaceuticals, try some antioxidants. Speak to your local pharmacist initially about remedies to relieve stress. There are various remedies that protect you from heart disease and lower your blood pressure.

7. 7.Afternoon naps can help. If you work from home, or are on the road a lot, find times in the day to relax this way. This is particularly effective if you tend to work irregular hours. This will make you feel more rested and generally more willing to face the day ahead.

Enforce these remedies to relieve stress each day to keep a healthy body and mind. Set a time that is convenient to perform the tasks, and stick to a schedule that works around your other daily commitments.

Don't let stress control you; it can only do that if you allow that to happen.

CHAPTER 8- REMEDIES FOR CONSTIPATION

Constipation is one of those things that no one really wants to talk about; yet everyone suffers from it at some point in their lives. Even though you may be embarrassed by this issue, chronic constipation is not only uncomfortable, it's also unhealthy. Before you run over to the local drug store to buy some sort of over the counter medicine to cure your next bout of constipation, you may want to consider the healthier alternative of constipation home remedies.

Most people know that their diet has a direct impact on having regular bowel movements. If your diet doesn't contain enough fiber you will likely suffer from constipation on a fairly regular basis. Just increasing your daily fiber intake can help prevent, or at least lessen, the amount of times you suffer from this issue.

Here are some other simple daily lifestyle changes you can make starting right now, that will help you greatly reduce the amount of times you have to suffer from constipation:

1. If you are already constipated try drinking a small glass of prune or apricot juice daily until you get back to normal. Then in order to keep yourself regular, you should drink a glass once or twice a week. Your body will let you know how much you need. If you don't like juice you can also eat the fruits, apricots or prunes.
2. It's also important to drink plenty of water every day. It may sound weird, but there are a lot of people in our country who are dehydrated, they simply don't drink enough water during the day. This can have a lot of negative effects on the body, and constipation is one of them. Drink more water.

3. Flaxseed can help you stay regular and can be stored in the refrigerator for some time. You can grind it up and keep it handy in the refrigerator. You can mix it in with a glass of juice or water or you can sprinkle it on top of your daily bowl of cereal.

4. Try to add some type of movement to your daily routine. Exercise has many health benefits and one of them is to keep your bowels working properly. Something as simple as a daily walk helps keep your digestive tract humming along.

5. There are herbal supplements available that will help you cleanse and detoxify your intestinal tract. Be careful before you use them though, and talk to your doctor about any possible interactions with medicines you are already taking.

These simple constipation home remedies can not only help you cure a bout of constipation but also help you prevent it from happening in the first place. Everyone suffers from constipation at one time or another, even if you eat right and get plenty of exercise, to lessen the frequency just remember to drink plenty of water, eat high fiber foods, take a fiber supplement, and keep moving. If you do that, everything else will stay moving the way it should too.

REMEDIES TO KEEP YOU REGULAR

Many people suffer with constipation and though it may appear to be an amusing situation for those looking in, for the person who has to live with this condition it can be a serious problem. Constipation home remedies are often the first port of call for someone who has constipation and with good reason; most of these home remedies work and work very well.

The symptoms of constipation can range from nausea, leg pains, headache, flatulence, fever and loss of appetite; all of which should

Mihalis Kapakolis

not be underestimated and can become problems in themselves. It should be noted at this point, that even if bowel movements are occurring, there could still be constipation. This is because if you have irregular bowel movements i.e. they do not happen every day and are easy to pass, you could also be considered to be constipated.

For virtually everyone who has constipation, their first port of call when looking for constipation home remedies should be to look at their diets. Plainly put if you put in the right amounts of foods, in the right amounts of combinations, then it should be easy to come out and that will limit the need for exploring further constipation home remedies.

Generally we should all aim to eat more fruits and more vegetables. This will add bulk and fiber to the diet and so help with relieving constipation. However, try to avoid those vegetables that are known to encourage flatulence: these include cabbage, sprouts, beans and foods such as nuts and also some dried foods. Processed, fatty foods and fried foods are also best avoided.

Instead one of the fruits that should be added to the diet is figs. Well known throughout time as one of the constipation home remedies, figs can be soaked overnight in water and be ready for breakfast the next morning. You can also use figs as the base for a homemade blended drink. Simply throw in three or four figs, add some oat milk and some prune juice and blend. This is a super drink that when taken regularly for several days will usually help to relieve constipation.

Wholegrain breads and cereals should also be added to the diet of anyone who has irregular bowel movements or is constipated. These breads and cereals help to add the necessary bulk that our bodies need to remove the waste. In the same way the fiber that these foods possess, is also vital to keep the bowels healthy and functioning.

Add exercise to your daily regime and drink plenty of water as this will help to keep your system working healthy and encourage the waste to naturally and easily leave the body.

CHAPTER 9- HOMEOPATHY REMEDIES

REMEDIES FOR ASTHMA

The term homeopathy owes its etymology from the Greek words that mean "suffering" and then "similar". In the world of homeopathy, the remedies are done by treating the ailment or disease with the ingredient or substance which has actually caused it. Let us put it this way, someone who suffers from allergens is given a miniscule amount of the same allergen for the purpose of immunizing him to it. Therefore, he will not have the same violent reaction in the event that he once again gets exposed to the allergen. The theory behind the homeopathy remedies is that these active substances motivate the human body's resistance to fight off these immune system invaders.

There are several homeopathy remedies for various diseases and illnesses. Asthma is only among the several lineups of conditions which can be covered by homeopathy remedies. Better know about it as it might help you in a lot of ways.

Among ten people, at least six of them are afflicted with asthma. Such is the case in several countries. In Latin, asthma is meant to refer to the process of breathing hard. As defined within the premises of medical concern, asthma is a type of chronic lung disease which is described by the spasm and inflammation of the bronchial airways or tubes. The bronchial tubes are those which act as the passageway of air in and out of one's lungs. In the case of asthmatic persons, their lungs get extra sensitive and generate too much reaction with irritants as compared to the individuals who do not suffer the ailment.

Those who are quite familiar with the homeopathy treatment are likely to wonder if there is a homeopathy remedy for asthma.

There are a number of homeopathy remedy alternatives for this kind of ailment. The medicines alone are unable to guarantee the everlasting cure for asthma but then homeopathy remedies could do great deals. Homeopathy remedies for asthma vary depending on its severity level. The use of homeopathy remedies actually reduces and eliminates the necessity to take in the inhalers and synthetic drugs for asthma. Typically, the patient will be advised to take natural herbs and to do away with the foods and other practices that may trigger the asthma attack.

As an integral part of the holistic approach adopted by homeopathy, the remedies for the ailment include the use of herbals and other natural medicines which do not in any way produce side effects that may harm the overall lifestyle of the asthma sufferer. In light of the homeopathy asthma natural medicines, other homeopathy remedies include the following:

1. Keep the bed and beddings clean at all times. The blankets and pillowcases should be washed with hot water.
2. Keep the pets out of the room.
3. Quit smoking or never go near someone who's smoking.
4. Maintain proper lighting and ventilation.
5. Homeopathy Remedies for Increased Libido

Most people, even the medical practitioners, have visualized the great effects and safety of the practice of homeopathy. This is due to the fact that not only homeopathy remedies are able to come up with wise relief for temporarily occurring or suffered disorders but they are as well able to give off a long-based healing term to an individual because of its holistic nature and approach. For most of its practitioners, homeopathy is regarded as a medication that has the power of leading a patient into full recovery from a certain disease and likewise provides a much better understanding regarding his situation.

The healing measure as provided by homeopathy is a lot easier and more secured that no further relapses are expected to occur in the near future. It is by the nature of the homeopathy treatment remedies that the body's natural defenses are roused to action so that the proper functioning of the cells will be met.

What are some of the common problems treated by homeopathy remedies? Homeopathic are made out by utilizing any of the remedies of mineral, plant, animal, or chemical substances. They are diluted in water and shaken vigorously. They become more effective when alternately diluted and then shaken sequentially. It is further advised that only miniscule doses are to be used. Among the homeopathy remedies are as follows:

The severe dose of the Ipecac will induce vomiting but the diluted dose of it is a homeopathy remedy for the control of vomiting and nausea.

Usually, the intake of coffee before turning in at night will cause you to be deprived of sleep yet with the miniscule dose of it; it becomes a homeopathic remedy for insomnia.

Diarrhea is likely to be provoked by the intake of a great dose of the sodium sulfate yet with the homeopathic advisable dose; it is able to treat the bowel disorder.

The intake of the homeopathy products that either delay the ejaculation or increase the libido for both men and women has been proven by some to be effective. This is in turn one of the most recent acclaimed homeopathy remedy for increased libido.

REMEDIES FOR INCREASING LIBIDO

If you fall under the category along with other couple who've been trying to conceive for months and even years, then you must see the underlying problem. It means that there is a pertaining defect with yours' or your partner's libido, sexual energy, or erectile ability. Losing the desire for intercourse is affected by a lot of factors. It could be the vices such as drinking and smoking, malnutrition, lack of bodily nutrients and minerals, and a lot others. These factors disable the proper production of sex hormones therefore making the intercourse less interesting and futile to the greatest length.

With this problem is a now known homeopathy remedy for increased libido. A particular homeopath, Dr. GR Anjum has concocted Spreme and Viagit Love Tonic as homeopathy remedy for increased libido. The Spreme is devised to delay ejaculation by means of the gentle desensitizing of the penis so that a longer span of lovemaking can be ensured.

The Viagit Love Tonic, on the other hand, is one natural-based homeopathy remedy for increased libido which then supplies more sexual energies in both of the couple.

These homeopathy remedy for increased libido products are made in Great Britain with the assurance that the quality is suitable enough to prove it effective even for the vegetarians. Now if you and your partner are confronted with the same dilemma, you know which homeopathy remedy for increased libido products to turn to.

THE REMEDY FOR BABY TEETHING

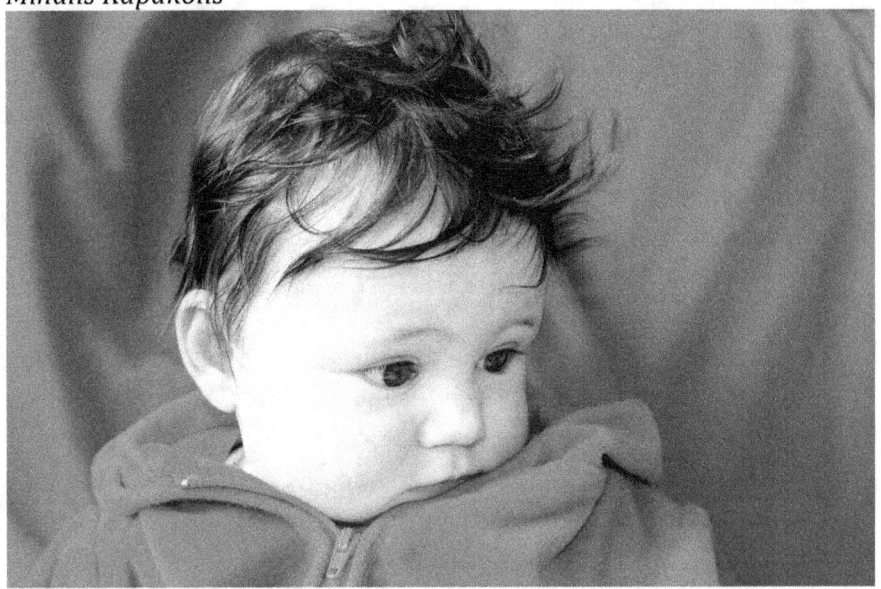

The growth of the popularity of homeopathy is undeniable. Homeopathy schools are continually increasing in number and it is likewise the same with the would-be homeopaths. In the United States alone, homeopathy schools are easily accessed whether the individual wishes to take the classes along with the others or to simply remain at home for online lessons. The homeopathy schools have with them a ready educational prospectus that will allow the student to learn the basics and the apt remedies for certain conditions.

Now in terms of baby teething, homeopathy schools are as well aware of the necessary remedies for it. Most of you pity the babies when they are ill. Why not? They are unable to speak for themselves. They cannot tell you what they exactly feel and how painful it is for them. The worst part is when the baby gets a fever alongside with the teething process. In the homeopathy schools, the best recourses for baby teething are discussed to you.

Nothing will be of too much relief to you if you see your baby smiling and enjoying despite his teething process. You may be intrigued to use the teething gel yet you can be better off with the homeopathy remedies. There is no doubt that the homeopathy remedies as taught in the homeopathy schools are effective, safe, painless, and non-toxic then you may be assured that your babies will be provided with the utmost relief.

There are a lot of homeopathy remedies that you can choose from. You have to remember though that some remedies work well with other babies whereas it may not have the same effect with yours. It is worth investigating to which homeopathy remedy your baby will react best. Remedies for Baby Teething:

The apis mellifica or whole honeybee. This is utilized to provide relief to the swollen gums. This remedy has been founded in the year 1835 by none other than Rev. Brauns from Germany. The remedy is easy to prepare.

The calcarea carbonica. Babies who are categorized as late or slow developers are more prone to suffering pain when teething. This homeopathy remedy is best for them especially if they find it hard to learn to crawl, walk, or if their heads usually sweat out during their sleeps.

The chamomilla. The remedy is best for babies who have swollen, reddish, tender gums, irritable, and hard to comfort except when being carried.

The oil of cloves. These substances are endowed with natural anesthetic factors. It can be given to the baby along with the organic oil of the sunflower.

The kreosotum. This homeopathy remedy is best in easing out the stress from the child during the teething period. The substance is best in hindering the possible decaying of the tooth.

The natural stick in licorice. It soothes the baby's painful feeling as the stick is chewed on.

The pulsatilla. This is good for babies who are often tearful, clingy, or nervous.

The silica or silicea. This is best for easing the difficult period of teething.

The sulphur. This homeopathy remedy is recommended for babies who likely develop rashes either on the chin or on the diaper area especially during those teething durations. Diarrhea can become the result of too much stress felt during this period.

Let your baby remain calm during the teething process. You can learn so much about the significant remedies from the homeopathy schools in your area.

Homeopathy often gets a bad rap among those who think modern western medicine is the only possible way of treating every ailment. But that doesn't really make sense when you think about it, does it? After all, modern medicine is a very new concept, yet human beings were able to survive for millennia without it. Homeopathy remedies work differently than other remedies. Instead of using something to counteract an ill effect, homeopathy will introduce a super-diluted form of it and then let the body send out its own natural defenses.

That's not as strange as it first sounds when you consider that many modern vaccinations work the same way. However, homeopathy takes it a step further and tries to find natural compounds that will cause the body to unleash its defense mechanisms.

While modern vaccines will use a weakened form of whatever disease they're trying to fight, homeopathy remedies can be derived from minerals, bark, roots, leaves, oils or just about any other naturally occurring substance. In some cases, ingredients that would otherwise be poisonous are used, though heavily diluted.

Another interesting difference between modern medicine and homeopathy remedies is that modern medicine tends to focus more on treating symptoms, whereas homeopathy seeks to fix the root of the problem. For example, if you have a cough then the medical establishment says you should take cough medicine to stop coughing. The problem is that your body is coughing for a reason; it's trying to get something nasty out of your system. So you may think you're getting better because you're not coughing, but suppressing a cough only keeps the nasty stuff in your body longer.

Mihalis Kapakolis

Homeopathy would also try to stop your cough, but not by suppressing it. The thinking is that your body needs to fight off whatever it is that's making it sick and the coughing is part of that process. However, by introducing the right (and heavily-diluted) compound, your body will unleash its natural defenses and actually cure the problem that's causing the cough.

Sticking to the same example, the funny thing is that you may cough even more by using homeopathy remedies, but that will only be temporary. In other words, you may actually feel sicker for a short while as your body does what it's designed to do, but once it's done, you will feel much better. Of course you can always take cough medicine that does nothing to treat the real problem, but why would you want to?

Modern medicine would scoff at this idea, but what it comes down is whether it works or not. There are surprisingly few studies into homeopathy because they just dismiss it without thought, and that's a shame. Whatever the case may be, it's hard to argue with the countless people who have felt better after using homeopathy remedies. So feel free to smile as the skeptics arch their eyebrows (as they keep coughing), you know what really works.

REMEDIES FOR CHILDREN WITH ADHD

Attention Deficit Hyperactivity Disorder is a condition that is marked by impulsive behaviors in children that is not caused by poor child rearing but because of certain genetic abnormalities that cause them to behave as such.

If you have ever encountered a child who runs in and out of the room and excessively roll on the floor without direction, you might have seen a child with ADHD. There are also those who daydream their days away without any sign of moving back to normal affairs and others could sit inattentively for a couple of hours straight. While normal children could display various symptoms that characterize ADHD, their behaviors could still is distinguished clearly. Nevertheless, symptoms of ADHD could be quite hard to distinguish as there are other conditions that display similar indications.

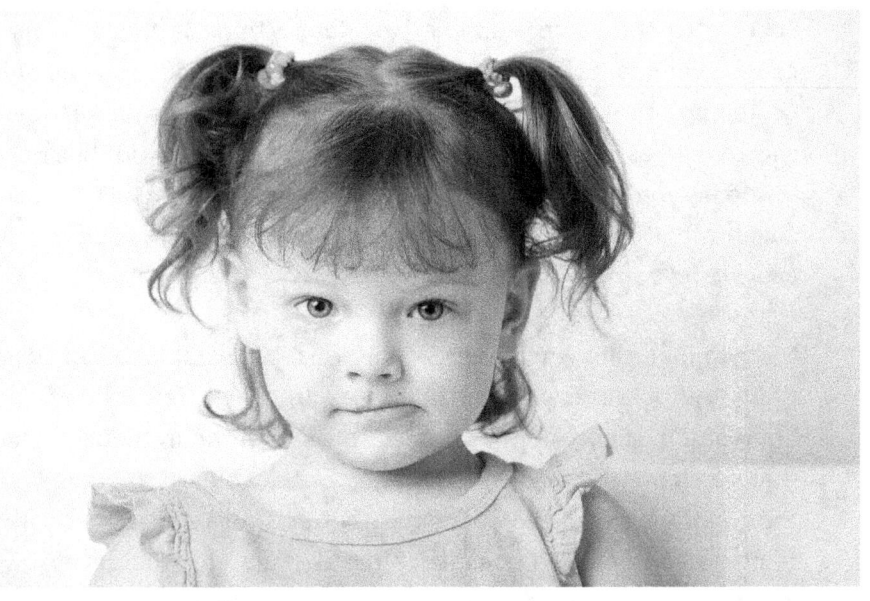

Normally, ADHD is treated with medications like oral antihypertensive, Ritalin and antidepressants. Even with careful observation and administration, side effects could still arise. Additionally, most drugs can't be recommended with children 6 years and below since many of them could have adverse effects such as toxicity. Lack of dosage could also affect the health of the child due to lack of proper measures that would determine the negative drug interactions.

Researches propose though of some proven homeopathic remedies for children with Attention deficit Hyperactivity Disorder that are effective in the treatment of disorder. Some of them are the following:

1. Anacardium: This is often recommended for children who feel isolated, put down, pathologically inferior, and separated from the world.
2. Argentums nitricum: This works specifically for those who have inner aggression that manifest through having sensations of an evil speaking to one ear and an angel speaking to another, for malicious and cruel patients and for those who act like they have no conscience.
3. Aranea ixabola: This helps treat children with fascination on spiders and those who excessively tease.
4. Baryta carbonica: This works for children with apparently delayed or arrested developments.
5. Baryta iodatum: This is indicated for patients displaying difficulty of concentration, restlessness, nervousness and canine-like appetite.
6. Belladonna: This homeopathic treatment is used for those who have the tendency towards poor learning, night terrors and associated conditions, and sensitivity to noises.
7. Bismuthum subnitricum: This treatment is used for children who excessively cling to their mothers or caregivers.
8. Calcarea phosphorica: This is recommended for children with symptoms such as dissatisfaction, frustration, restlessness, shyness, and fussiness.
9. Cannabis indica: This homeopathic remedy is indicated for children who have space disorientation, inattentiveness, and confusion, has the fear of going insane, with de-realization, and has problems with attention.
10. Ferrum metallicum: This is given to children who have sluggish mind and have difficulty in recollecting memories, for those who have anemia or frequent headaches and those who display particularly strange like or dislike on tomatoes.

11. Gallic acidum: This is given to patients who display dislike with their loved ones.

12. Hyoscyamus: This is a homeopathic remedy for children with difficulty on controlling impulses, excessive talking with manic episodes which can result to hitting or screaming, with depression after each episode.

13. Stramonium: This is proven for children with violent and fearful nature. Those with extreme hyperactivity and for those who tend to have fast, loud and incoherent speech.

These are just some of the proven homeopathic remedies for children with ADHD. For safer use, you could consult your child therapist so as to prevent any adverse effects.

CHAPTER 10- AYURVEDIC REMEDIES

Ayurveda is a holistic approach to health that has been around for centuries and is now gaining in popularity after having been largely forgotten for hundreds of years. Ayurveda promotes a healthy lifestyle where you keep your body in balance and if an illness does occur you don't just treat the symptoms, which is what most Western forms of medicine do, instead you attack the underlying cause of the problem so you can have a permanent fix to the problem. There are ayurvedic home remedies for many types of common illnesses.

Ayurvedic promotes a balance between the three energies that promote inner and outer health. These energies are called doshas and everyone has their own unique balance of doshas. Finding out your natural balance is part of determining the best ayurvedic remedy for you and your situation.

There are herbal Ayurvedic remedies for many diseases of the nervous system, lymphatic system respiratory system, digestive and circulatory system. As you can see, there is a lot of different common medical issues that may be able to be resolved using this ancient knowledge.

Make sure, though, that before you start any type of alternative medical regime you talk to your doctor first. Don't make the mistake of thinking that just because these are natural herbs that they are completely safe. There can still be negative side effects when you combine some herbal remedies with over the counter or prescription drugs you may already be taking.

It's also important that you learn what you are doing and what part of the plant you need to use such as the roots, the leaves, or the stems. You also need to know exact quantities to use as well as the exact way to prepare the herb; if you choose to do it on your own, be willing to spend some time learning more about the various herbs and how best to utilize their power. This isn't something you should try to do without carefully learning how to do it properly.

It's also important to note that when you are using natural herbal remedies that they will generally take longer to work than other forms of medicine. This is actually a good thing since unlike many other drugs which only mask the symptoms, think of a cough drop, the natural remedies will actually help you fix the underlying cause. Even though it may take longer the result should be more permanent than when you just take a drug to mask the symptoms so you can feel better.

Before you go out and buy a lot of herbs to make your own ayurvedic home remedies you should consult with an Ayurvedic practitioner. There is a definite method to this practice and you don't want to start taking a lot of herbs if you don't know what the overall effect will be on your body. Take some time and find an expert in your area who can show you just what you need to do to get the maximum benefit from this form of medicine.

CHAPTER 11- REMEDIES FOR IRRITABLE BOWEL SYNDROME

When it comes to finding relief from IBS, irritable bowel syndrome remedy, you actually have many products to choose from. The trick is to find the product or combination of products that will work well for you and your unique set of symptoms. Some will work for some people but not others; it's often a case of trial and error... as frustrating as that can be. The good news is that you shouldn't give up, just keep looking until you find the product(s) that can help relieve your symptoms.

The most common symptoms of IBS are diarrhea, abdominal pain, cramping and bloating. These symptoms can also be caused by other illnesses which can be ruled out by various tests and procedures your doctor recommends.

If you suffer from frequent bouts of loose stool then you may have IBS with diarrhea. If you have less frequent but harder bowel movements you may be suffering from IBS with constipation. It can vary from one instance to another, at times you may have diarrhea and at others constipation. This is one of the reasons why it's so tough to provide effective treatment for IBS. The symptoms can always be changing so the medications needed for relief will have to change as well.

If your symptoms include diarrhea your best options for some relief would be over the counter anti-diarrheal medicines, if you suffer from constipation you'll need laxatives to help provide you with some relief. Many irritable bowel syndrome remedy will work fine for the short term but shouldn't be taken for extended periods of time.

Outbreaks are sometimes triggered by eating a food that didn't agree with you. If you can identify which foods you are sensitive to you may be able to cut that food out of your daily diet. This one simple step can be an effective irritable bowel syndrome remedy

Stress is another thing that tends to trigger outbreaks. Getting rid of stress from your life (as much as possible) can help cut back on the number of outbreaks you get and it can also improve your overall health. It's been proven that too much stress can contribute to heart disease and high blood pressure as well. Finding ways to cut down some of your stress can help you maintain good health overall, not just alleviate your IBS symptoms.

Some patients report that using heating pads or hot baths can help relieve some of the cramping that comes with an outbreak. Using yoga or meditation to help you relax has been proven to help many people get some relief from their IBS symptoms too.

If you ever find yourself suffering from symptoms you suspect may be IBS your first step should be to see your doctor. He can diagnose you and prescribe some medications that may help you find a little relief.

Finding effective remedies for IBS might seem like a daunting task, but it's not impossible. Just keep looking until you find the irritable bowel syndrome remedy, or combination of things, that will work for you and give you some much needed relief.

REMEDIES

You can hear from any person that the illness can be quite irritating and you will feel absurd. This is mainly due to the truth that though the disease is not dangerous it cannot be cured easily. The symptoms also greatly affect the routine life of people who suffer.

Mihalis Kapakolis

As personal life is also affected people seek remedy for it and try to find different treatment for the syndrome to help regulate the symptoms of it.

For each person each treatment is required as the treatment depends on each and even their efficiency can vary.

ALTERNATIVE THERAPY

According to the proof, studies have found out that the stress and mental life has got a great impact on Irritable bowel Syndrome. This is possibly the reason by which alternate treatment is preferred by people. Alternative therapy comprises of several remedies like Ayurvedic, Homeopathic, yoga etc., all of which are not related to Allopathic.

Some of the examples are as follows:

a) Acupuncture .It is one of the best types of alternate solution to the Irritable Bowel Syndrome. This is mainly due to the fact that practitioners of this solution cure this illness on a case to work format.

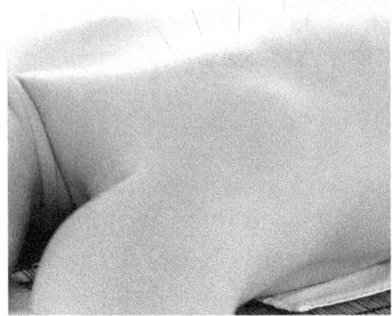

The working of acupuncture on Irritable bowel syndrome is by trying to free up the obstructions in a person's life energy. This is exercise by pinning needles on various portions of the body .The patient need not worry as the needle used will be so thin and will only reduce the ail caused by the IBS symptoms.

b) Yoga-As told, the stress has a heavy effect on symptoms of Irritable Bowel syndrome. Many people switch on to yoga to keep their mind relaxed, calm and eliminate stress in their work life as well as personal life .Though yoga doesn't have any direct effect on Irritable Bowel Syndrome; the treatment is quite appealing as the person will be in a relaxed state which supports the cure.

c) Ayurvedic-we all are behind old herbs which were used as medicine, as they do have much side effect and also cure naturally. Ayurveda has begun to play a major role in the treatment of Irritable Bowel Syndrome. Treatments are done on one by one basis. A person need to tell the Ayurvedic doctor, what he is suffering from and the doctor will cure him accordingly by giving a mixture of herbs which will help.

Mihalis Kapakolis

d)Medical-In order to assist them with the syndrome ,Irritable Bowel Syndrome is much easier to people. It's also widely relied on because people accept it more, as they understand them more.

There are two kinds of medical treatment available for Irritable Bowel Syndrome

a) Medicines/Drugs- people who suffer from this type of irritable Bowel Syndrome are given prescription drug of several medicines, often the drugs are used to reduce the pain caused, act as a stabilizer for the digestive process and even help in decreasing depression. Only a blend of drugs will help in treating this syndrome

b) Counseling-Many people go for advice or consultation from a doctor which is the best method of treating oneself having Irritable bowel Syndrome. People who are having such symptoms often worsen them by thinking constantly about it. Mental/Emotional counseling is supposed to work out well and it can be considered as part of treatment of this syndrome.

CHAPTER 12- REMEDIES FOR DETOX AND WEIGHT LOSS

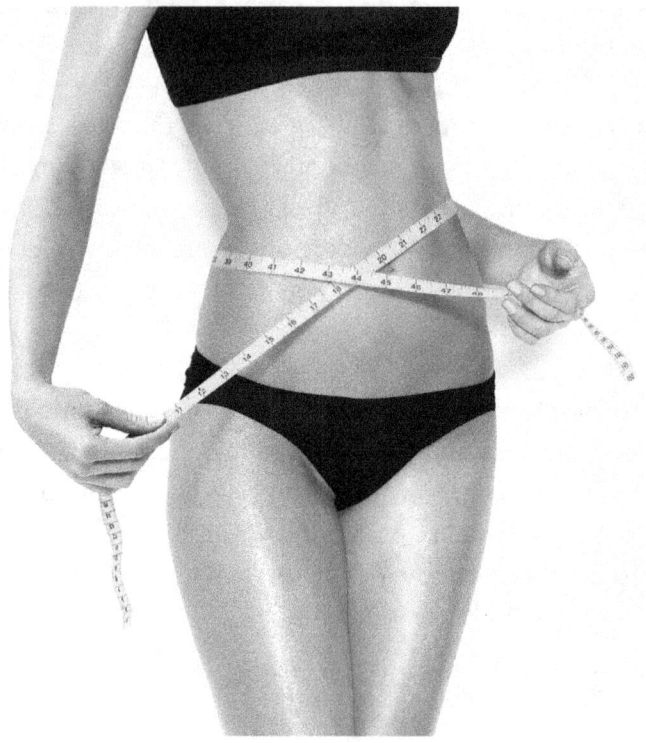

DETOX

The accumulated toxins inside your body must be cleared in order for it to function well. Your body needs to be healed to regain energy. There is one effective way of clearing your body from these unwanted toxins and it is called body detox or body detoxification using natural herbs. However, it is not taken as a single step but a continued process so that the natural ability of your body is supported for the effective dispelling of toxins every day.

Another process being incorporated in body detox together with using herbs is limiting the toxins which enter your body. Eliminating or restricting the use of the usual culprits such as refined sugar, caffeine, alcohol, tobacco, drugs, household chemicals, and petroleum or synthetic-based body paraphernalia is a very good way of starting.

You should start eating organic natural diet foods, getting regular exercise, and drinking adequate amounts of water to facilitate your detoxification. Your body can adjust easily in a gradual change that is much better compared to other practices.

The following herbs that have known to be effective for many years can be used as a home remedy. These are the natural way of body detoxification.

1. Psyllium seeds and husks contain high fiber which can gently act as a natural laxative. You can utilize it by soaking the seeds in water. Psyllium is generally considered as adaptogenic which supports the healthy function of your bowel. It is also useful in treating diarrhea and other irritable bowel diseases. It is a very good choice for body detoxification since its gelatinous substance after soaking absorbs toxins.
2. Hydrangea root and the Joe pye weed (gravel root) helps in preventing, dissolving, and expelling stones and crystals in the bladder and kidneys. It is good to keep your kidneys free from any obstructions to stay in good working condition essential in effective elimination of toxins.
3. Cascara Sagrada is used also as natural laxatives. It could be safe even for longer duration of usage where it strengthens your colon's muscles.
4. Alder buckthorn's barks are also used but it must first be dried and be stored for at least one year since its fresh barks are so strong which can be considered toxic.

5. Juniper berries also promote the urinary system's overall health. It detoxifies and strengthens your urinary tract, bladder, and kidneys. It is excellent for cleaning purposes but prolonged usage is not recommended because it can cause some overtaxing in your kidneys.

6. Nettles also have detoxifying properties which can be extended not just in your urinary system. Nevertheless overusing it can display similar effects as the juniper berries.

7. Burdock seeds and roots are similar to nettles. It has mild and cleansing diuretic action but has stronger effects. Heavy metals inside your body can be removed by using burdock.

8. Basil, cypress, celery, grapefruit, lemon, fennel, rosemary, thyme, and patchouli contains essential oils effective for flushing out toxins underneath your skin and stimulating circulation of your lymph.

9. Dandelion root and milk thistle help in cleansing and strengthening your liver. Milk thistle has silymarin which does not only protect your liver but helps in regenerating itself. Dandelion root helps in removing waste products from your gallbladder and kidneys.

You would never have any problems if your body needs detoxification at home. You can try using these wonderful herbs to obtain their natural remedies. Rejuvenate yourself and feel good about it.

CHINESE WEIGHT LOSS TEA AS A DIET REMEDY

Chinese weight loss tea uses natural products to help you achieve the slimmer body you desire. There are a variety of different types of Chinese weight loss tea including WuLi, Pu-Erh, and Oolong tea.

After water, tea is the most widely consumed beverage on earth. So, can tea actually help you lose weight and achieve your ideal body?

It is easy to incorporate tea into your diet. In fact, one of the best things about Chinese weight loss tea is that you are adding something rather than subtracting something from your diet.

The Chinese weight loss tea works by acting as a metabolic stimulant. It helps your body to burn more calories and fats by increasing bodily functions. Because it has only four calories a serving, you will not be gaining any weight when you drink tea of any kind. However, when you drink Chinese weight loss tea, you take in phenols which help to burn fat and decrease blood cholesterol levels.

Chinese tea that helps you lose weight will have up to 70 percent oxidation. This speeds up your metabolism and activates enzymes to let you burn fat.

If you are drinking Chinese tea with the intention of losing weight, you must drink it at least two times a day. The rest of your diet should be healthy as well. You should include some physical activity in your daily regime as well.

Tea must be grown in a region which receives at least 50 inches of water per year. Tea has a growth phase and a dormant phase. When the new tea shoots emerge as the weather begins to warm, the plant can be harvested. All types of tea come from the same plant and are harvested in the same way.

But it is the drying process that gives some teas their special weight loss effects. There are some teas that are dried for up to 100 years! (That is long term planning!)

Most of the tea plant evaporates in the drying process. Most of the time, the drying process involves baking the tea leaves.

After the tea is dried, there may be a final process known as curing which gives tea its great flavor.

Chinese weight loss tea is oxidized for two to three days and is known as blue tea or semi-oxidized tea. It tends to taste more like green tea than black tea.

Chinese weight loss tea is best prepared with very warm, but not boiling, water. You can brew this tea several times from the same leaves. The taste actually improves with each brewing. It is common to steep the tea up to five times and the consensus is the third brewing is best.

If you want to get skinny, one of the tools at your disposal is Chinese weight loss tea.

CHAPTER 13- REMEDIES FOR ALLERGIES

Millions of people suffer from allergies. There are all types of allergies, everything from dust and pollen, to animal dander, to certain types of foods. The most common symptoms of an allergy are a runny nose, watery itchy eyes, sneezing, pressure, headaches, and nausea. The good news is there are many very effective allergies home remedies that you can use that will eliminate, or at least diminish, your reliance on expensive and side effect heavy prescription and over the counter drugs and may help you get rid of the allergies altogether.

Here are some things that you can try:

1. Taking Vitamin E is believed to help increase your body's ability to fight off allergens. Many people have gotten relief from their allergies by taking a daily dose of Vitamin E.
2. Many people claim that adding a few drops of castor oil to a half cup of juice can help alleviate your allergy. You can also add the castor oil to a glass of water if you prefer.
3. Use the allergy relief furnace filters in your furnace and make sure to replace them as often as the manufacturer recommends.
4. Use a bleach water solution in any areas of your home that tend to get damp. This can help eliminate the growth of mold which is a prime cause of allergies.
5. Keep your pets bathed and brushed. If you can't do it yourself take them to a groomer.
6. Try to avoid any house cleaning chores that tend to stir up a lot of dust. If possible get someone else to vacuum, dust, or sweep.

7. If you can, try to replace your carpets with wood or tile flooring and just a few area rugs. Carpets are like magnets and they can really hold on to a lot of dust and dander.

8. Buy an air purifier and make sure to replace the filters frequently.

9. Keep your pets out of your sleeping area. This is the one area of your house that it's particularly important to be an allergy free zone. You need to be fully rested and if you're up sneezing all night long you can't get the sleep you need.

10. Make sure to frequently wash all of your bedding in hot water. This is another place that dust mites and dander can really build up fast, and since this is also where you sleep it's very important to keep it as free of dust as possible.

11. When cutting the grass you should consider wearing a mask to keep the dust from blowing into your face. This may also help whenever you are out working in the yard if you are prone to seasonal allergies.

Whether you are looking for something to relieve your allergy symptoms or eliminate your allergies altogether, these allergies home remedies can provide you with some much needed relief. Use one, or all, of the tips on this list and keep looking until you find the combination that works best for you. You do have options and don't have to just rely on store bought allergy products.

CHAPTER 14- REMEDIES FOR FLU AND BRONCHITIS

FLU REMEDIES

Unfortunately none of us are immune to getting sick, especially in the winter when we spend more time inside spreading germs back and forth to one another. If you have the flu and want to get over it as soon as possible, who wouldn't? Then here are some simple flu home remedies that should help.

Of course, if you're vomiting and/or have diarrhea to the point where you can't keep anything down you may want to visit your doctor. There are some nasty flu strains going around and even if the flu you have is just a 'normal' seasonal flu, it's still easy to get dehydrated which in itself can be dangerous. Better to be safe than sorry.

In the meantime, try these simple remedies so you can start feeling better sooner:

1. If you are suffering from a sore throat a good remedy is a saltwater gargle. All you have to do is add about a teaspoon of salt to a glass of warm water and mix. Take a large amount in your mouth, don't swallow it, and gargle. Repeat a few times. Make sure you don't swallow the salt water because that can upset your stomach even further. You can do this several times throughout the day.

2. To ease your sore throat and calm your stomach you can use a blend of herbs to make a tea. Mix bayberry bark with ginger root in the following amounts: 1 teaspoon of bayberry bark, 1 teaspoon of grated ginger, and 1/2 teaspoon of cayenne

powder and add to 1 cup of boiling water, allow it to steep for about 30 minutes than enjoy.

3. There are many homemade cough syrup recipes you can use, for now try this one: take two parts elecampane root , two parts marshmallow root, and one part horehound root, mix altogether and cover with honey. Let stand in a warm area of your home for about 24 hours. Strain the mixture and take syrup as needed, about a teaspoon at a time.

There are many other types of cough syrup and tea recipes that can help you feel better when you are sick. You may want to try different recipes to find the ones that you like the best: have the best flavor and work well for you.

And of course if you want to prevent sickness keep stocked up on some things that will help keep your immune system strong: Vitamin C, garlic, cinnamon, and honey to name a few. You can also add some fresh lemon juice to warm water and drink it daily to keep your immune system in tip top shape.

Hopefully you can escape the cold and flu season unscathed, but if you do catch some nasty bug use these flu home remedies. Not only can they help you feel better sooner, you can save some money on all the expensive over the counter medications. You're already sick; you don't need to make it worse by having a big bill from your local drug store!

HERBAL REMEDIES FOR BRONCHITIS

There are mainly two kinds of bronchitis. One is the acute bronchitis, and the other is called chronic bronchitis. Bronchitis is an illness where the bronchial tube is inflamed due to viral infection.

Mihalis Kapakolis

Acute bronchitis is usually caused by a virus infection. However, there are some cases where bacteria and fungus infection can also cause bronchitis. You have to consider that you need to know about bronchitis in order for you to know how to treat it properly and also know how to manage it. Acute bronchitis is considered to be very easy to treat and manage. This kind of bronchitis will usually last for only 10 to 12 days and will also be followed closely by flu or cold. Acute bronchitis will contain the following signs and symptoms that you need to be aware of:

1. Mild chest pain
2. Hacking cough with mucus
3. Mild fever
4. Headaches
5. Sinus congestion
6. Squeezing sensation around the eyes
7. Wheezing sound when breathing
8. Fatigue
9. Chest discomfort

These are the signs and symptoms of acute bronchitis that you should know about. It is important that you should consult your doctor immediately after you feel the mentioned signs and symptoms. They will be able to know what kind of infection you have or whether it is a viral, bacterial or fungal infection. With a proper diagnosis, the doctor will be able to give you the right kind of medicine.

Bronchitis caused by viruses doesn't usually need medications, but you can consider taking medications for symptom relief, such as nasal decongestant, and anti-inflammatory drugs. Again, you first need to tell your doctor about your intentions of taking some medications as you may have allergies in certain kinds of drugs and some drugs are also considered too dangerous when combined, especially in pregnant women.

Today, research has found that some herbal medicines can help in alleviating the symptoms of bronchitis. One kind of herbal medicine that can help alleviate coughing associated with bronchitis is eucalyptus oil. Eucalyptus oil helps loosen the phlegm to make it easier for the lungs to get rid of the mucus secretion inside. In fact, inhaling eucalyptus has been recommended by a lot of medical practitioners all over the world for bronchitis patients. To prevent bronchitis, or to at least minimize the chances of getting bronchitis, eating a lot of garlic is recommended. Garlic is filled with chemicals that kill virus and bacteria. In short, garlic is a natural antiviral and antibacterial herb.

Recent studies have found that the stinging nettle plant can treat bronchitis and other kinds of respiratory illnesses. The juice inside the roots and leaves mixed with honey or sugar can relieve the signs and symptoms that you can suffer from bronchitis.

Plants containing a good source of vitamin C can also help prevent and alleviate the symptoms of bronchitis. It is also recommended that you should eat plants containing magnesium as this can also help in alleviating the symptoms of bronchitis.

These are some of the herbal remedies that you can consider using if you have bronchitis. You can also try boiling oregano leaves and drink the juice.

It is recommended that you should not disregard if you are already seeing the early signs and symptoms of acute bronchitis. You have to remember that if you neglect it, it make likely develop into its chronic form that will cause permanent damage to your respiratory system.

CHAPTER 15- REMEDIES FOR THE LIVER

Your liver is essentially the filter for your body and keeping it healthy using liver home remedies will help make sure that you stay healthy or can get healthy. If you think of the air filter for your car and all the things that get trapped in it just from driving around, you might get an idea of how your liver looks. Your air filter has to be able to allow clean air to run through your car to help it keep peak performance. When it gets clogged up your car won't work as well. Your liver acts in much the same way and using liver home remedies will help you get and keep your body at peak performance.

Your liver acts as a filter for your blood. It takes all the impurities that your body has absorbed and filters them out so that your heart can keep pumping right. The toxins get into your bloodstream through a few avenues. It gets in through digestion, respiration, and the skin. What it filters out is viruses, bacteria, and other things that act as poisons to our bodies. The liver's job is to get these things out of our bloodstream before it has a chance to do some damage to us. It detoxifies our bodies by filtering the blood.

The liver also helps filter and detoxify the body by creating bile that is necessary for proper digestion. It also changes the toxins into a form that is easily removed from the body through urine or stools after it has also neutralized or decreased the potency of the toxins. The liver has to be helped so that it can run smoothly making your body run smoothly.

Many liver home remedies, that you will find can keep that filter running well, use different foods such as certain fruits and vegetables.

Mix fresh papaya juice with lime juice and drink it with some regularity. For those who have cirrhosis of the liver mixing tablespoon of papaya juice with about 10 drops of lime juice and taking it twice daily. This has been shown to be one of the better and more used liver home remedies.

Carrots are also known to provide some great cleaning benefits for your bodies filter. Mix carrot juice with spinach juice and possibly cucumber juice and beet juice to help also with other liver problems including cirrhosis of the liver.

One of the most powerful among those foods that are liver home remedies is the cabbage. It aids the breakdown of toxins in the liver and helps reduce the congestion that takes place in the liver.

Another thing that is going to be the biggest part of keeping your liver clean is using water. Water is great at flushing out the impurities and should be drunk frequently.

Your liver is one of the hardest working and most important parts of your body. Do what you can to make sure that the filter is healthy and is able to do its job by taking advantage of these liver home remedies.

As always, it is always prudent to consult with your professional health care provider, to make sure there is no conflict between the home remedies and any medications you are taking.

CHAPTER 16- APPLE CIDER-HEALING REMEDIES

Many of the healing home remedies that have been used by people for generations and even going back thousands of years has involved vinegar. The father of modern medicine, Hippocrates (from whom the Hippocratic Oath came) used to prescribe it for persistent coughs. He was also understood to have used it and prescribed it mixed with honey for energy and general well-being. Ever since then it has been used to treat many ailments and considered and seen as part of many healing home remedies.

Apple cider vinegar has been used to treat such things as acne, asthma, helping control blood pressure, reducing cholesterol. There are many other uses that could be found as well. Many of them revolve around making an apple cider vinegar tonic which is adding 2 or 3 teaspoons to 8 ounces of water but there are also many other ways that it is used as well.

One of the healing home remedies for helping reduce acne blemishes is apple cider vinegar. Taking a solution of vinegar to water, much like what is used in the tonic; apply to your face a couple times a day using a cotton ball. This will not only help cut down infection, but it will help dry out inflammation.

One of the ways that apple cider vinegar is considered one of the better healing home remedies is in helping to treat asthma. There are people who have, with success, drank the tonic and applied a compress soaked with vinegar to the inside wrists.

To help control blood pressure apple cider vinegar is being used as one of the good healing home remedies. A tablespoon of apple cider vinegar and a tablespoon of honey in a glass of water a couple times a day will help lower blood pressure. Both apple cider vinegar and honey have high potassium levels which helps balance sodium levels in the body. The vinegar also has magnesium which helps relax blood vessel walls which also helps lower the pressure.

Another way that it is used is reducing cholesterol. It has water soluble pectin in it that helps absorb cholesterol and fat and helps eliminate it from the body. The amino acids in it help cut down and neutralize LDL cholesterol. Cutting down on the bad fats, increasing the amount of fiber you take in and using the vinegar tonic will help significantly drop your cholesterol levels.

In no way should any of this be used instead of what your doctor may prescribe for your ailments but there is little doubt that these healing home remedies using apple cider vinegar will help other treatments you have to give you better overall health.

CHAPTER 17- REMEDIES TO HELP WITH MENOPAUSE

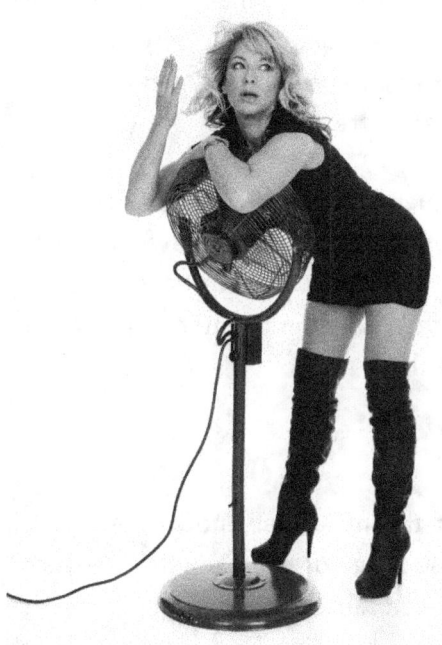

Menopause marks the end of a woman's child bearing years. It is the time when she stops getting periods, and for many women that is a good thing. Unfortunately, it isn't that simple. The process can take years from beginning to end and there are unpleasant symptoms, but you can get natural remedies to help with menopause symptoms.

Every woman is different and will go through menopause at different ages, for different lengths of time and with different levels of discomfort. If you are one of the unlucky ones who have fairly severe symptoms and / or they last a long time, you may be able to use natural remedies to help with menopause.

There are many possible symptoms of menopause and not every woman will have every one of them, and the ones you do get may not be severe, but for each symptom of menopause, there are some herbal remedies that may offer some relief. Here is a list of some of the most common menopausal symptoms and the herbal remedies that are commonly used to treat them.

Before you start taking any supplements of any kind, though, make sure you discuss possible interactions you may have with your doctor. Even all natural herbal remedies can have dangerous side effects and interactions with other over the counter or prescribed medications. Make sure you ask first.

OK, as promised, here they are:

1. Hot flashes. This is one of the most well-known menopause symptoms and it can run the range of being a mild annoyance to so severe that you can't even function. It's about much more than just getting hot. It's about feeling like you have a high fever along with sweating, headaches and nausea. Two of the most common herbal treatments for hot flashes are Black Cohosh and Red Clover. There are many women who swear by one or the other of these herbs to cut back on the frequency or severity of their hot flashes. Whether or not you will get relief remains to be seen but as long as you won't have any interactions with your other medications, you might as well give it a try to find out for sure.

2. Anxiety and insomnia are also very common side effects of menopause. There are two popular herbal treatments for these symptoms: Ginseng and Kava. Both have shown to be helpful

with anxiety and mood swings during menopause, but Ginseng has also been shown to help with sleeplessness.

3. Other things that may provide relief for one or more symptoms of menopause, or at least maintain your overall health during this period are: Vitamins A, D and B complex, Calcium, Evening Primrose Oil, Wild Yam, Licorice and St. Johns Wort.

Also staying healthy by eating right drinking plenty of water and staying active can also help keep your body healthy during this challenging time in your life.

Even though these remedies are all natural that doesn't necessarily mean that they don't have any side effects. Always talk to your doctor first before you start using any natural remedies to help with menopause.

CHAPTER 18- REMEDIES FOR YEAST INFECTIONS

You will never know what can be very useful in your kitchen. Just a little flick of your hand, your basic ingredients and seasonings may become an effective medical kit which can remedy injuries like simple cuts and get rid of infections like yeast infections. The microorganisms Candida albicans, causes yeast infections. But don't be surprised to know that home remedies for yeast infection can be very effective in getting rid of those microorganisms.

Candida is a kind of microorganism that is always present in our body. When its environment, including our body, changes the growth of the fungi suddenly increases which causes the infections. This change in the environment may vary from acid and alkaline imbalance to poor nutrition. Some triggers also include an increase intake of sugar, changes in the body's hormones, antibiotics, and even birth control pills. Any one of these or combination of these factors can trigger the proliferation of the fungi resulting to infections bringing with it the problems of itching, burning, irritation, and the presence of white or yellowish discharge.

Although a number of products are commercially available to help soothe the discomfort brought by yeast infection, you might find these products a little expensive or buying them would be quite inconvenient or you need the remedy this instant. Also, there might be a chance that the fungi develop a resistance to commercially available medicines.

Some of the remedies that have been recommended include the use of borax especially if the yeast infection causes discharge that looks like egg white; calcarea carbonica to help with the itching and burning sensations felt before and after menstruation; kali bichromicum to remedy a very uncomfortable discharge with itching and burning; natrum muriaticum; pulsatilla; sepia; and sulphur.

You can fight microorganisms with other microorganisms. We're talking about the use of probiotics which are friendly microbial organisms that occur naturally in the digestive tract and vagina. The growth of probiotic microorganism suppresses the growth of the Candida which cases the infections. It's a battle of microorganisms.

There's a big chance that these remedies are not readily available in your homes. There are natural and more homemade remedies that are available to you.

Garlic has been found to be effective by some people when it comes to treating yeast infections. What you can do is get a couple of garlic cloves and smash and convert it into paste. You then apply that garlic paste around the vagina area. The antibacterial properties of garlic can help in getting rid of those pesky fungi. The only setback would be the smell.

A not so smelly alternative would be the use of honey. However, the smell may not be as strong as garlic but the stickiness of honey would be quite uncomfortable. Nevertheless, according to testimonials applying honey on the affected regions helps alleviate the various symptoms of the infection. You apply honey and leave it for about 30 minutes before rinsing with warm water.

Another good antibacterial and antifungal remedy would be vinegar. Vinegar mixed in warm water is said to be quite effective. You need to soak the area for at least 20 minutes though to see and feel some effects. Cider vinegar is said to be more effective.

Home Remedies Bible

These are but a few of the home remedies for yeast infection. There might be a couple of others that you might heard of but before you decide to use them, it would be best to ask around or read more about them to make sure that you won't be doing more harm than good.

CHAPTER 19- REMEDIES FOR VARICOSE VEINS

If you have varicose veins and are looking for varicose veins remedies to help lessen the discomfort that they can cause, I have a few suggestions for you. There are several things you can do some with advice of your doctor and some you can just do on your own, that can help lessen the discomfort and even prevent varicose veins from developing.

Talk to your doctor and ask if you are healthy enough to start a walking program. Walking improves blood circulation in your legs. Talking to your doctor first is important so you do not cause yourself other injuries. Get yourself a good pair of walking shoes before you start, too. Your feet and legs will thank you.

Losing any and all excess weight is another one of several great varicose veins remedies you can do and will take the pressure off your legs and help decrease the severity of your varicose veins. Walking will help with losing the weight and if you combine the exercise with a low salt, high fiber diet you will also help decrease the edema, or swelling that goes along with varicose veins. Talk to your doctor first before starting a diet plan.

Low heeled shoes are best to wear when standing for long periods of time or walking they work your calves better. Standing or walking in high heeled shoes shortens the calf muscle therefore decreasing the blood flow and varicose veins and possibly pain or discomfort. Loosen up the clothes you wear, too. Do not wear tight clothing and steer clear of girdles or body slimming undergarments; they can cut off circulation to your lower body.

If you have a job where you have to sit or stand for extended periods of time, try to take a few breaks during your day and elevate your feet and lower legs above the level of your heart. This will not only help with blood circulation but will take some pressure off and decrease what's called dependent edema (swelling of the lower legs, feet and ankles).

Also get up and move around, do not sit at your desk for hours on end, move around for five or ten minutes every 30 minutes to an hour to keep the blood moving. If you have to stand for extended periods, bend your knees, stretch out a little, or do some deep knee bends to keep the blood moving. Doing these simple exercises when you are at work will not only help with the varicose veins but they will help keep you alert on the job, too.

One last thing you can do for yourself when trying to control varicose veins is, do not ever sit with your legs crossed. Think about it, when you sit with your legs crossed for an extended period of time, does your foot fall asleep? This is a circulation issue and should be avoided at all costs. Crossing your legs when sitting will cut off the circulation in your lower legs increasing the likelihood you will develop varicose veins later in life. Prevent varicose veins by not crossing your legs when you are sitting.

If any of these suggestions for varicose veins remedies do not help relieve the discomfort you are experiencing, speak with your doctor about other treatment options available to you.

This article is for information purposes only and is not professional medical advice. Nor should it be used as medical advice at any time. You should consult with your own Physician or other proper medical professionals prior to determining treatment or diagnosis.

CHAPTER 20- REMEDY AGAINST THE SPREAD OF BED BUGS

Bed bugs are tiny oval shaped wingless creatures. They are about four to five millimeters in length that you can hardly see. Bed bugs used to crawl, but it is noteworthy that they are swift runner among other insects. Bed bugs are dark brown in color and become reddish when they suck blood. It is hard to find them on brown flooring or furniture but they can be easily seen on white and light surfaces. They are so tiny and have thin body formation that can squeeze and fit easily in minute cracks and gaps. You will seldom find them at open areas; mostly they are used to hide themselves in small splits in the home furnishing.

There are two main kinds of bed bugs that bite humans and animals. The first kind is of common bed bugs also called as cimex lectularius. Large numbers of them are present in Australia. This kind is commonly present in any nocks and cranny; they spread and breed in areas that meet their nourishment requirements. Second kind is tropical, also known as cimex hemipterus. These are called tropical bed bugs because, according to medical entomology department, these bed bugs are supposed to live in tropical areas in the past.

Bed bugs are not only breed and distribute in homes, bird's nests etc. but also found on human and animal body. These habitats are most suitable for bed bugs because of the warmth which is the ideal place. Moreover, these places provide them favorable conditions to breed and multiple in numbers. They act as predators and feed on their host i.e. warm blooded animals. It is worth mentioning that bed bugs never distribute consistently throughout the environment. When the environment is unfavorable, they used to distribute in harborages like cracks and crevices in walls, furniture, wood walls, wall units, carpeting and wall papers. Moreover, they also distribute on trees and their leaves and roots.

Bed bugs are habitually more active during night. But, they also attack and suck their predator's blood when they are hungry during day time. In homes the warmest place is the bedroom which ensures the presence of bed bugs. More precisely they are present the one place where humans sleep i.e. the bed! Their existence in bed rooms gave them the name of bed bugs.

Bed bugs also live and distribute on cloths. It is interesting to note that bed bugs do not remain attached to the fur or feathers; they leave their host as soon as their hunger is satisfied. They are also found in mattress, bed cover, blanket, bed casing, under carpet, behind wallpapers and so on. The proper precautions must be taken to reduce the existence and spread of bed bugs. There are many insecticides and pesticides available in market which do not only kill bed bugs but also kill their eggs and give you peace of mind.

CHAPTER 21- PREVENTION: HOME REMEDIES CAN KEEP YOU HEALTHY

Are you tired or afraid of getting sick? Prevention home remedies are highly sought after and used by those who want to avoid getting sick. They can be things that you learn to avoid, things that you have to force yourself to change in your lifestyle, or things that you have to learn to eat or drink.

Much of learning to prevent disease revolves around having a healthier lifestyle. If you are overweight, your overall health will improve dramatically as will your chances of staying healthy. Exercising is going to be a huge part of prevention home remedies because not only does it help you lose weight and take pressure off your heart, it strengthens all of your body and helps get rid of the toxins that are in your body.

Eating right is a big part of getting and staying healthy. Like above, it will help you lose weight but it will also help ensure that you are putting good things in your body to fuel it and help get rid of the toxins that are in your body.

One of the tougher things to do, as if the above wasn't already tough enough, is limiting your intake of alcohol and cutting out smoking. Both of those are proven to weaken your body and will cause you to have severe and avoidable problems down the road. Lowering your blood pressure by de-stressing is something that will help other prevention home remedies and actually could be considered one itself. Finding ways to avoid stress and unwind will help keep your body from getting sick. The more your mind stresses, the harder it is on your body. Find ways to rest and relax. Get out of incredibly stressful situations if at all possible.

Two of the best prevention home remedies are getting lots of sleep and drinking lots of water. Your body needs to have about 8 hours of good sleep per night. The less sleep your body has to go on, the more stressed it gets.

If your body gets too stressed it becomes very susceptible to sickness and disease. When that happens you are going to probably find yourself in bed much longer than you would like or can afford. You should also drink more water. Drink water when you wake up and before you go to bed. Drink water at each meal and in between meals. Try to keep from getting thirsty; if you get thirsty you are already dehydrated.

Other things that are prevention home remedies are simple things like washing your hands frequently, especially when touching things that could have viruses on it (which is pretty much anything that people touch). Clean those items when you can especially when they are in places that you frequent or live in.

Get yourself on a good vitamin regimen to help ensure that your body is getting the nutrients it needs. Make sure that you are also getting enough fiber in your diet to help get rid of toxins in your body. Most of these things are common sense but it is amazing how often common sense ceases to be common in our own lives. Taking these measures will help us realize that the best and most effective prevention home remedies are not that difficult to find and that it really is easy to stay healthy.

CHAPTER 22- HOME REMEDIES CANCER CURES DO THEY EXIST?

Many people who are trying to find some way to fight cancer want to know if there is some home remedies cancer cures available. This is because they don't want to go through the treatments that can make you almost as sick as the cancer itself. Many people have opinions on this matter and it should be discussed with the team of professionals treating you as well as getting input from family who is battling with you. Cancer has to be attacked on many different fronts but even then it is a very tough adversary that has claimed millions of lives.

For every home remedies cancer cures you hear about, you need to research. One may be out there that works for some people but not enough to consider it a true cure. Sometimes it will work in conjunction with other treatments that are going on and will result in remission. Sometimes all you can hope for is to find some home remedies cancer treatment that will help you endure the treatment going on. Even with that, you need to check with your team of physicians to see if there would be any negative interaction with treatments that you are undergoing.

Some of the home remedies cancer treatments you will find would be good for helping prevent cancer. Garlic is one of the things that can really help you get healthy or at least healthier and make your body stronger to withstand cancer. Garlic is proven to be a very strong antibiotic that will stimulate the white blood cells effectiveness as well as T cells.

It can help improve your immunity which, because of cancer treatments, may be compromised. It has been shown in clinical studies to prevent and, according to some, help cure some forms of cancer. It may be tough but taking a clove or two of garlic daily, either chewing or just swallowing with water, may help increase your rate of getting or staying healthy.

Garlic and turmeric both have shown to have the ability to block tumor nourishment and help starve them or stunt their growth.

For the nausea and vomiting that takes place many times after chemotherapy, a homeopathic remedy may be cadmium sulphuratum. This can be found at many wellness stores or bought online. It is pretty affordable.

Some of the foods that one eats will help prevent or fight cancer and are capable home remedies cancer fighters. Tomatoes are known to help with lung cancer as well as cervix cancer, throat cancer, and prostate cancer. Raw red cabbage will help as will cooked beets because of the flavanoids present. Spinach would be another helper because of the richness in anti-oxidants such as vitamins C and beta carotene.

There are many options available to help fight cancer or at the very least help prevent cancer. It will take a bit of research on your part and a lot of asking and working with those who are working with you. Be sure that you are going to be able to find things that are home remedies cancer fighters.

As stated several times throughout the article, you should consult with your professional health care provider; to determine if there would be any conflict with your regular medical treatment.

CHAPTER 23- HOME REMEDIES OR SURGICAL METHODS

The remedies available in the market today to remove moles, warts, and skin tags vary in terms of effectiveness. A certain remedy may work for one individual but it may not work for another. Perhaps the most effective method to remove moles, warts, and skin tags is through surgical methods. This is usually done in the clinic or in the hospital by a competent and qualified doctor.

The method is somehow painful because some methods employ local anesthetic while other methods employ general anesthetic. Moles, warts, and skin tags can occur in the different areas of the body. These skin lesions are commonly found on the face, hands, knees, and feet. Oftentimes, by employing the surgical methods, a scar is left behind. This is the main reason why some individuals resort to herbal or home remedies because they don't want to end up with a scar that will always remind them of the skin lesion; not only that, home and herbal remedies are readily available at home and you don't need to spend huge money unlike the surgical methods.

Another consideration is the pain felt during surgical removal of moles, warts, and skin lesions. Some individuals are scared to undergo any surgical method because they don't want to feel pain. The home and herbal remedies will not make them feel uneasy because the remedies are not painful except in the case of plantar warts. Plantar warts are found on the soled of your feet. The plantar warts are quite painful especially if you're treating them but the pain is tolerable. By choosing the home and herbal remedies, you still need to be aware of the possible risks.

Some individuals cut the skin lesions using scissors. This can be done but extra care should be observed. The scissors or any other cutting device should be sterilized to avoid infection and bleeding. You don't have to make a big fuss about your skin lesions because you can easily remove them without undergoing any surgical method. One effective way to remove the skin lesions is by tying a string around the lesion.

Leave the string in place for day and you will notice the mole, tag, or wart turn bluish in color. When the skin lesion turns black, you can wait until it falls off or you can snip or cut it off. The blood supply is cut because of the tight knot and so the skin lesion eventually falls off. Did you know that by opting for the doctor's solution the skin lesions are removed by using sharp blades and scissors?

If you're scared of blades and other sharp devices, you can stick to the natural remedies. There are various herbs that you can use to remove the skin lesion however it could take a couple of months before you can remove them completely. You need to apply the herbs everyday for several times and you must do this religiously; otherwise, you won't be able to rid your skin of the unsightly lesions.

According to some researches, there are some theories which explain how the moles, warts, and skin tags occur. Some studies even show that women are more prone to such conditions as compared to men. As you get older, you're more prone to these unwanted skin lesions. Simply practice good hygiene everyday and when you notice any skin lesion treat them immediately.

About The Author

Mihalis Kapakolis is an accomplished researcher who has done years of extensive studies in the areas of Health, Wellness and Natural Remedies for common ailments. With his Wealth of knowledge, Kapakolis has compiled this in-depth book which documents all the basic remedies which the reader would need to alleviate or treat a wide array of common medical conditions including: Asthma, Back Pain, Arthritis, Menopause and even ADHD in children.

In this book the author outlines various methods of treating these and other complaints using herbs and other items that can be found in most homes.